TOWARDS A SOCIOLOGY OF CANCER CAREGIVING

T0239825

For Anton, Colleen and 'Shrimp'

Towards a Sociology of Cancer Caregiving
Time to Feel

REBECCA E. OLSON
University of Queensland, Australia

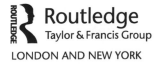

Routledge
Taylor & Francis Group

LONDON AND NEW YORK

First published 2015 by Ashgate Publishing

2 Park Square, Milton Park, Abingdon, Oxfordshire OX14 4RN
52 Vanderbilt Avenue, New York, NY 10017

Routledge is an imprint of the Taylor & Francis Group, an informa business

First issued in paperback 2020

Copyright © 2015 Rebecca E. Olson

Rebecca E. Olson has asserted her right under the Copyright, Designs and Patents Act, 1988, to be identified as the author of this work.

All rights reserved. No part of this book may be reprinted or reproduced or utilised in any form or by any electronic, mechanical, or other means, now known or hereafter invented, including photocopying and recording, or in any information storage or retrieval system, without permission in writing from the publishers.

Notice:
Product or corporate names may be trademarks or registered trademarks, and are used only for identification and explanation without intent to infringe.

British Library Cataloguing in Publication Data
A catalogue record for this book is available from the British Library

The Library of Congress has cataloged the printed edition as follows:
Olson, Rebecca E.
    Towards a sociology of cancer caregiving : time to feel / by Rebecca E. Olson.
        pages cm
    Includes bibliographical references and index.
    ISBN 978-1-4724-4659-6 (hardback)
1. Cancer–Patients–Care. 2. Cancer–Social aspects. 3. Caregivers. I. Title.

    RC262.O48 2015
    616.99'4–dc23

                                                                    2015004258

ISBN 978-1-4724-4659-6 (hbk)
ISBN 978-0-367-59890-7 (pbk)

Contents

Acknowledgements

This book is the culmination of nine years of researching and publishing on informal cancer caregiving. Over this time, many contributed. While the work is my own, and I take responsibility for its contributions and faults, it would not have been possible without the moral, financial and intellectual support provided by so many generous people.

Most of all, I am indebted to the participants, many of whom were time-poor, for sharing their inspirational stories so articulately and openly. I am thankful for the financial support provided by Cancer Australia and Cancer Council ACT (CA-A 0708/56) which made this research possible. The University of Western Sydney also provided the study leave from teaching required to make this book possible and for that I am very grateful.

I would like to recognise staff at the Australian National University for their guidance during data collection and analysis, especially Associate Professor Kevin White and Professor Dorothy Broom. Thank you Dr James Connor, University of New South Wales, Canberra, for helpful feedback on earlier drafts and for permission to extend our co-authored work here as Chapter 4. I am also grateful to colleagues at Victoria University of Wellington, Associate Professor Annemarie Jutel, Professor Kevin Dew and Dr Allison Kirkman, for their reflections and hospitality during the drafting stage.

Preface

The idea of hearing a cancer diagnosis for my partner sounds almost as difficult (albeit different) as receiving the diagnosis myself, linked as it would be with the sense of a newly-limited term to a relationship I would have otherwise imagined (or at least hoped) unlimited. But I am reminded by the lyrics of *Iron and Wine*:

> One of us will die inside these arms
> Eyes wide open, naked as we came
> One will spread our ashes round the yard.
> (Beam, 2004)

Of course it's unlikely that we will shuffle off our mortal coil at the same time, so one will always 'die inside these arms'.

Tussling with the idea of our own mortality is hard to conceptualise; imagining a world without our life partners is as well. While we know our lives and those of our loved ones *will* end, we do not usually have a clear sense of how that end will occur. The cancer diagnosis, linked as it is to prognosis, brings that mortality into harsh reality (although cancer is not always synonymous with death, a fact that is often forgotten in the presence of the generally-feared diagnosis).

The cancer diagnosis is anchored in the popular imagination as proxy for a death warrant. We refer to it euphemistically in popular culture, as the 'Big C', a word so terrifying we are loathe to utter it. While there is no one cancer, but many; no pre-determined prognosis, but many; no one cell type, but many; to learn that one, or one's partner, has cancer is to endure a shock. The cancer diagnosis has the power to transform; even if there is no material change in an individual's condition; putting a name to a disease alters one's life story (Blaxter, 2004; Frank, 1995; Bury, 1982; Fleischman, 1999). Suzanne Fleischmann (1999: 10) wrote of her own diagnosis (which was to result in her untimely death):

> If a person is told 'you have cancer' (or any life-threatening disease) *these words* irrevocably alter that person's consciousness, view of the future, relationship with family and friends, and so on. Moreover, the utterance marks a boundary. It serves to divide a life into 'before' and 'after', and this division is henceforth superimposed onto every rewrite of the individual's life story.

Even when we're talking about a 'good' cancer, one with a high probability of survival, the phenomenological experience of the person with cancer becomes paced by the disease and its impact, rather than by previous markers such as relationships, accomplishments, and occupations.

The transformation, as this book demonstrates, is clearly not endured by the person with the diagnosis alone and Olson brings into stark relief the experience of people who accompany their spouses down the often-tortuous path of disease, sometimes towards remission, sometimes towards death. Historically, it was often they who would be told the cancer diagnosis instead of the patient; they were a kind of shield to protect the sick person, concealing the disease from their loved one. Nineteenth-century medical students were instructed in this practice: 'Whenever death lowers over the case, and you are solicited by anxious friends to reveal the imminent danger of your patient, decline, unless your patient makes a direct appeal to your candour' (Harrison, 1844: 10). There was less concern about how to protect the spouse.

But to think that this task of shielding the patient is without consequence for the spouse would be a mistake, as Olson highlights in the up-coming pages of this book. Diagnosis can wreak havoc on the carers, transforming their lives as well as those of the spouses for whom they care. Priorities shift, emotional expectations swing and relationships morph. As 'Matthew' (who will be introduced at the start of Chapter 4) describes it, following his wife's diagnosis of breast cancer, he now needs to show a new face, assume a different role. He tries, he says, to 'keep on this brave face ... be positive and be a pillar, the father, the head of the house' (p. 75). Being a caregiver is to become someone different: to learn a new idiom, take new initiatives, shoulder a greater burden in the partnership, and often, lose the support of the life partner one might have learned to rely upon.

It also casts a certain pall over the future. Not only are the cancer patient's prospects suspended, postponed or abandoned, so too are those of their caregivers. The future becomes uncertain. Caregivers in these pages describe living for the now, postponing future plans. This liminality gives rise to a mix of emotions for the carer. But, as they are not themselves facing death, their needs are often misunderstood or subordinated. They often have no way of telling their story, which becomes a kind of subtext to the main plot in which their spouses play the leading role.

This book foregrounds contemporary spouse carers of cancer patients, aiming to improve awareness and recognition of the existential and practical challenges of caregiving. Using methodological tools from sociology, it makes both practical and theoretical contributions. While it is written primarily for sociologists, it will be accessible to a wide audience. Grounded in spouse carers' stories, the book draws readers into both the difficulties and the opportunities that cancer diagnoses present. It will be of interest to carers wishing to reflect on their own and other carers' journeys and to clinicians seeking new ways of thinking and communicating about caregiving.

Just as this book was going to press, Richard Smith, former editor of the *British Medical Journal*, created a furore by suggesting that dying of cancer was the best way to go: 'You can say goodbye, reflect on your life, leave last messages, perhaps visit special places for a last time, listen to favourite pieces of music, read loved poems, and prepare, according to your beliefs, to meet your maker or enjoy eternal oblivion' (Smith, 2014). While his words are, self-admittedly, romantic, they do underline, despite all the challenges outlined above, the opportunity offered by dying from, or caring for, a partner with cancer. After a cancer diagnosis, the couple may have the time to resolve old disputes, say what needs to be said, and come out of the oblivion of the end in which they otherwise operate.

The opportunity is not lost on Olson's respondents and analysis. On page 83, we can see the words of Judy, who describes the changed relationship with her husband:

> We are like a pair of silly old idiots. We go for a walk in the evening holding hands. We never used to do that ... We [sit] out in the dark on the veranda and we [talk] about the past ... it [is] just lovely.

Similarly, on page 97, Joe speaks about how important it was, as a carer for his wife 'just to be able to lie together and hug each other'. He would wake up in the night whenever she stirred in order to be able to reposition her in the bed, something her paralysis prevented her from doing herself. For Joe, being able to hug his wife brought him emotionally closer to her, made him more settled within himself, and undoubtedly brought comfort to his wife.

These stories punctuate the *possibilities* that cancer presents for the caregiver, possibilities that are not necessarily, as Rebecca Olson reveals in this detailed field work, what caregivers experience (and this may just explain why Richard Smith was demonised for suggesting that a cancer death was a 'good' death). What is it that makes the experience of some cancer carers rewarding and others so burdensome? As we will see in the pages that follow, this is an important question, grounded in so many different areas. To provide a semblance of order in this morass of identity and emotion, of expectation and of uncertainty, we must first understand what is taking place, founding Olson's insistence that we cast a sociological gaze on the caregiving journey.

Important issues such as diagnosis, identity, social support, emotions, and indeed marriage, are social phenomena through which individuals attempt to map their pathways. Emotions in particular are a profoundly social process. By using a sociological approach, we can develop a means of describing and bearing witness to the 'cancer carers' unique experiences of loss, providing validation and potentially helping carers to feel less alone' (p. 121).

Understanding the experience of caregiving is imperative to strengthening the cancer caregiver/cared-for dyad. The wan 'it must be so hard!' is of little help, and, as this sociological inspection of caregiving reveals, there are many concrete issues at play that should be explored in order to provide a means of communicating both to and about the spouses' experience of caregiving.

The sociological framework used in this text provides ways of considering the realisation that 'One of us will die inside these arms' (Beam, 2004), ordering the social, cultural and temporal dimensions of the caregiver's experience. Under this light, we can adopt different ways of communicating about the emotional experiences of the carers of a spouse with cancer. We can find ways of legitimating the carer's role. And, we can begin to explore what political, financial and economic pressures contribute to, or detract from, what is potentially one of the most significant events in a couple's life together.

Associate Professor Annemarie Goldstein Jutel, RN PhD

Introduction

On one of the last warm days of autumn I entered a house on a quiet suburban Australian street. A soft-spoken man, Ian,[1] let me in. Pictures of him with his wife and children looking close, happy and satisfied with life hung on the walls. But, these were moments from the past. His home appeared to be weathered and worn both inside and out. The garden was overgrown, the open garage door revealed stacks of boxes and piles of toys. The interior was in a similar state: books overflowing from shelves and a carpet in need of vacuuming.

I was there to interview him about his experiences as a carer for his wife when she had cancer. As we began our interview it became clear that he too had seen better days. He told me how severely his wife's initial cancer diagnosis and subsequent recurrence had affected him and their relationship. Anxiety and depression had taken a crippling hold on his life. Every day he fought with his fear that his wife may die and he may have to raise their children alone. This fear had been affecting his work and his relationship with his wife. Her physical scars were a constant reminder of their mortality. Ian said, 'it's quite the loss …. From the aesthetic point of view, it reminds you of the, you know, possibility … it reminds you of the dangers you are in'. His fear and anxiety made it difficult for Ian to care for his wife, forcing him to rely on his wife for emotional support when he wanted to be providing her with emotional support.

> I didn't react as well as I should have … I was a bit of burden on her … [and my wife] felt somewhat under supported … she would sort of say that I was measuring the grave … which is not that helpful.

This was a source of guilt and embarrassment for Ian. Clearly, cancer had had a psychosocial impact, not just on his wife, but on Ian, her husband, and their entire family.

This book examines the impact of cancer on carers of a spouse with cancer. Caregiving has been the focus of an increasing number of studies and academic books over the preceding decades. Studies, using psychological scales, show caregiving to be a stressful and burdensome experience, especially for younger female carers (Li et al., 2013). Recent books articulate the social, cultural and historical changes in ethics, demographics and policy that have produced current forms of caregiving in western countries (Fine, 2007; Glenn, 2010; Hochschild, 2012; Bruhn and Rebach, 2014a). In this book I examine an important element

---

1   To protect the confidentiality of participants' identities, all names are pseudonyms.

of caregiving that often goes unseen in psychological and macro-sociological studies: carers' lived experiences. I narrow the scope further, to the lived experiences of carers of a spouse with cancer. In working towards a sociology of cancer caregiving, I examine the impact of recent social and policy shifts on the patterns of care, identities, relationships and emotional experiences of spouse cancer carers. This leads me to demonstrate that cancer caregiving is a process shaped by social, emotional, temporal, political and economic realities.[2] Thus, it is a topic that requires in-depth sociological inquiry.

Giving Care

Informal carers or caregivers are the friends or family members who provide informal physical and emotional support to a patient at home without pay (Blum and Sherman, 2010; Given et al., 2012). The changes in mood, function and behaviour that come with diseases such as dementia, stroke and cancer often necessitate assistance from an informal carer (Aubeeluck and Buchanan, 2006; Blum and Sherman, 2010). Carers' responsibilities include: direct care tasks (e.g., symptom management and assistance with mobility); indirect care tasks (e.g., coordinating appointments and communicating with health professionals and family); as well as emotional and social support (Given et al., 2012; Given et al., 2006).

Giving care, however, is more than the emotional and practical activities required to sustain another person. It is a complex act that emerges from a past relationship (Cash et al., 2013: 659). Unlike the formal caregiving performed by nurses and other health professionals, being an informal or family carer often stems from *caring about* the person in need of help with activities of daily living.[3] *Caring about* reflects concern for and 'feelings of responsibility for' the person in need of care (Glenn, 2010: 186). *Caring about*, or a past relationship with a person needing care, can prompt a would be carer to *care for* – that is to carry out the many activities of 'providing for the needs or well-being of another person' (Glenn, 2010: 186). Thus, caregiving is more than an activity; it is a relationship (Cash et al., 2013; Bruhn and Rebach, 2014a), and one that is increasingly commonplace in our ageing societies. With improvements in diagnosis and survival rates, the number of informal cancer carers has increased (Sinfield et al., 2012). Informal carers are now the primary source of community care (Burns et al., 2010; Stetz and Brown, 2004). In Australia, for example, 12 per cent of the population is involved in some form of caregiving (ABS, 2013).

---

2 See Kleinman (2012), who argues that these are central features of the 'art of medicine' more generally.

3 Cahill, however, points out that 'caregiving can and does take place in the absence of love and affection, so it cannot be assumed that love is the underlying motivation behind duty to care' (Cahill, 1999; cited in Cash et al., 2013: 670).

In the United States of America (USA), the figures are higher at 29 per cent of the adult population (Bruhn and Rebach, 2014b).

Informal or family carers are usually close relatives, spouses (40 per cent), parents (20 per cent) or children (25 per cent) (Duckett, 2004), who perform practical and medical tasks for a patient such as help with shopping, transportation, hygiene, cooking and treatment administration (Given et al., 2012; Given et al., 2006; Kleinman, 2012). It is also a very emotional role, with patients identifying carers as the people with whom they 'share' their illness journey (Thomas et al., 2002: 539). Carers' experiences vary across diagnoses, relationships and time (Greenwood et al., 2009; Blum and Sherman, 2010; Molyneaux et al., 2011; Sjolander and Ahlstrom, 2012; Cassidy, 2013; Li et al., 2013). Overall, carers describe challenges that are: 1) physical and technical, with carers required to lift and administer medications; 2) administrative, with carers required to coordinate care across multiple health and support service systems; 3) emotional, with carers often mourning the social death of their family member before the physical death; and 4) social, with the demands of caregiving often eroding into other life domains (Soothill et al., 2001; Funk et al., 2009; Greenwood et al., 2009; Williams et al., 2009; Li et al., 2013; Olson, 2012).

Caregiving can also be detrimental to a carer's health (Chambers et al., 2001). More specifically, it has been found to impact on carers' finances, physical health and mental health. Carers often suffer financial losses with nearly two thirds (58 per cent) of all primary carers outside the labour market, compared to less than one third (31 per cent) of the wider Australian population (ABS, 2013). In the USA, the costs associated with providing care are similarly high, with nearly fifty per cent of working caregivers reporting depleted savings due to caregiving expenses (Bruhn and Rebach, 2014b).

Caregiving can also have a detrimental impact on a carer's physical health. In addition to being relied on to carry, transfer and physically support another adult, which can injure a carer's musculoskeletal health (Evandrou, 1996), many carers also have pre-existing health problems (Thomas et al., 2002).[4] Caregiving takes time away from salutogenic activities such as physical exercise (Li et al., 2013; Toseland et al., 1995). Furthermore, a carer's reduced income can have a negative impact on their physical health. Evandrou (1996) points out that a lower income when another family member's medical bills are overwhelming[5] may push a carer to leave his or her own medical problems unaddressed.

---

4 Thirty-five per cent of cancer carers in Thomas et al.'s (2002) study had pre-existing health problems.

5 For example, Sharon (50s, spouse with neurological cancer), who had been a carer for her husband off and on for almost twenty years, said caregiving and cancer had had a noticeable impact on their finances. 'The life we have had has been different ... because we have had not much money ... we haven't had a lot of overseas holidays or trips or anything because most of our money has gone on expensive scans every three months. Rather expensive operations. So a lot of medical bills have accounted for a lot of our money'.

Multiple studies show that caregiving is a mentally and physically tiring role with carers suffering from higher rates of neglected health problems, major depression, anxiety, panic attacks and stress than their non-caregiving counterparts (Hodges et al., 2005; Northouse et al., 2000; Weitzner et al., 2000; Li et al., 2013). The psychosocial toll is often worse for carers. When compared with the cancer patients in their care, carers often have greater levels of distress, anxiety and unmet psychological needs (Thomas et al., 2001; Hodges et al., 2005; Northouse et al., 2000). Quantitative studies show that being younger (under 65), female and caring for someone in the advanced stages of disease is statistically associated with higher risk of burden and anxiety (Gallicchio et al., 2002; Burns et al., 2004; Chiou et al., 2005; Given et al., 2012; Li et al., 2013). Yet, it is important to note that not all caregiving is perceived as 'burdensome' (Greenwood et al., 2009). Many carers find the role fulfilling, growing closer with the care recipient (Mutch, 2010; Williams et al., 2009; Blum and Sherman, 2010; Cassidy, 2013). Kramer (1997), for example, found that some dementia carers feel a greater sense of importance and satisfaction in their lives as a result of their caring responsibilities.

The negative financial, physical and mental health impacts that caregiving can have make caregiving an important topic for sociological study. Providing further support for its sociological investigation is the prevalence of the role – it is one we are all likely to be called upon to perform at one or multiple points in our lives.[6] The uncertainty, fear and grief associated with a *cancer* diagnosis makes cancer caregiving an especially important subject for sociological inquiry. To begin this inquiry, let us start by locating current forms of caregiving in history, place and policy.

Historical Contexts of Care

Caregiving is a feature of human life. Families have historically been, and still are, responsible for providing care to their young, old and incapacitated (Bruhn and Rebach, 2014b; Blank and Burau, 2014). The form of caregiving that now prevails, and the current social organisation of care, however, is relatively new (Glenn, 2010). Advances in public health and medical technology have extended life expectancy. Political shifts – namely growing neoliberalism – along with an aversion to institutional care have moved care from the hospital to the home in countries with advanced economies. But, the ideologies around who is responsible for care – families or the state – and whether and how family carers should be

---

6   USA President Jimmy Carter's wife Rosalynn famously declared, 'There are only four kinds of people in the world – those who have been caregivers, those who are currently caregivers, those who will be caregivers, and those who will need caregivers' (Carter and Golant, 1994: 3; cited in Bruhn and Rebach, 2014b: 9).

supported differ across Organisation for Economic Cooperation and Development (OECD) countries.[7]

Throughout much of humanity's long history, most deaths were sudden with little if any period of disability before death (Kellehear, 2007). Famine was a frequent concern and it was not uncommon for pandemics of infectious diseases to kill off large portions of a population (Beaglehole and Bonita, 2004). While occasional periods of illness and injury required support from family, life was short and medical interventions were simple.

The late nineteenth and early twentieth century saw increased affluence and food security, along with the acceptance of germ theory. Subsequent changes to hygiene, water treatment, housing, vaccination and public health programmes in developed countries have led to dramatic increases in life expectancy (Szreter, 2002; McKeown, 1979; Baum, 2008). Medical and surgical interventions have also improved. By the end of the twentieth century, diseases like cancer and even HIV were no longer synonymous with death (Sontag, 1991).

Life expectancy has increased significantly. While a child born in Australia during the 1880s could expect to live 47–50 years, a child born in the 2000s can expect to live to between 79–83 years old (ABS, 2011). Life expectancies in the United Kingdom (UK), Japan and USA show similar trends (The World Bank, 2014). Today, the end of life in most developed countries is characterised by chronic illness and a two to four year period of disability, not to mention intermittent periods of illness throughout the preceding decades (Wilkinson, 2006). These demographic changes mean there is a greater need for care.

During the nineteenth century, periods of convalescence and recuperation were spent at home, under the care of family and a local physician (Bruhn and Rebach, 2014c; Bella, 2010). The family's – most often the women's – responsibility to care was not only a reflection of patriarchal ideologies of the time; in many instances it was also a social policy of the state and a legal requirement. In her book *Forced to Care: Coercion and Caregiving in America*, Glenn (2010) shows how institutional, ideological and political forces converged in the USA over the course of the nineteenth and twentieth century to anchor women and minorities with unpaid or low paying caregiving responsibilities. These forces were enacted through, for example, reform schools for imprisoned women in sewing, cooking and other forms of domestic labour. Through these and other socialisation projects, the state imposed an American ideology of women as housekeepers and reinforced a woman's 'obligation to care' (Glenn, 2010: 87). Furthermore, this care work was defined, not as labour, but as love (Glenn, 2010; Bruhn and Rebach, 2014d). Judicial rulings related to will disputes during the twentieth century enforced this familial ideology of care as 'natural'. Individuals who agreed to provide care for

---

7   An overview of the contexts of care across all nations and cultures could fill a book in its own right and is thus outside the scope of this book. The focus here is limited to a brief outline of the historical and political contexts of caregiving in a select number of developed countries.

a person who was incapacitated in exchange for a bequest who then married the care receiver, were regularly denied any claim to financial compensation. In a famous case from the USA state of Kentucky, *Foxworthy* vs *Addams* (1910), the judge ruled that:

> It is the duty of husband and wife to attend, nurse, and care for each other when either is unable to care for himself. It would be contrary to public policy to permit either to make an enforceable contract with the other to perform such services as are ordinarily imposed upon them by the marital relations, and which should be the natural prompting of that love and affection which should always exist between husband and wife. (Court of Appeals of Kentucky, 1910; cited in Glenn, 2010: 98)

By the mid-twentieth century, the professionalisation of medicine and nursing had occurred and many caregiving responsibilities had been shifted from private homes to hospitals and other institutions (Bruhn and Rebach, 2014d). Health professionals and administrators depicted hospitals as superior environments for patient care because of improved sterility, technology and facilities for diagnosis and disciplined treatment of serious illness (Glenn, 2010; Bella, 2010). Diseases such as tuberculosis (Roth, 1963) and mental illness were treated on a long-term, inpatient basis. Hospital care followed a 'total' care and paternalistic model (Goffman, 1968). Care of patients with serious illnesses rarely took place at home.

The decades following World War II mark a period of significant improvements in medical technology and political change. Universal health care coverage was introduced in the UK, Canada and Australia (White, 2006; Bella, 2010; Duckett and Willcox, 2011). There was an ongoing feminist movement (Oakley, 1985), and individuals were re-conceptualised, from in need of protection, to self-sufficient during Reagan and Thatcher-era politics (Opie, 1992; Bella, 2010). The format and approach to providing medical care in Australia and many other countries subsequently changed from institutional and paternalistic care to community-based and family care.

This shift, from family-based care to institutional care and back again, is the consequence of multiple converging forces (Wyatt et al., 2010; Bella, 2010). One impetus was the growing sentiment that hospitals are too 'impersonal' (Little, 1995: 2). The cold interactions in institutions detailed in exposés such as Goffman's *Asylums* (1968) motivated a desire for more personalised and holistic patient care. Viewing economic and caring motives as discordant, de-institutionalisation and independent living movements gained momentum (Glenn, 2010; Kleinman, 2012). Many patients now prefer to be cared for by a family member at home (Johansson et al., 2011).

An increasing dislike for paternalism in medical interactions provided a second force behind the move from hospital to home (Salander and Moynihan, 2010; Duckett and Willcox, 2011). In eras past, medical practitioners were instructed, for example, to withhold 'the truth' about a patient's prognosis if it was 'not good for him [or her]' (Salander and Moynihan, 2010: 116). The public began questioning practices of withholding information from patients and allowing patients little say in their treatment (Surbone, 2006). An increasingly well informed public, with access to the internet, formed consumer groups, took legal action and demanded they be more involved in patient care (Turner, 2006).

The need to reduce costs associated with health care, however, arguably provided the strongest incentive for health care reform. An ageing population and declining birth rates, along with increasing specialisation and medical technology have steadily pushed up the cost of medical services (Blank and Burau, 2014; Gauld, 2009). In the USA, shifting care from hospital to home has been an important means of reducing labour costs to expand the profitability of the private health care system (Glenn, 2010). In countries with universal health care systems, such as Australia, it has been a means of containing costs (Davis and George, 1993; Duckett, 2004) to preserve the (relative) equity in access to health care that has become an ethical and political imperative (Little, 1995; Turner, 2006).[8]

In many developed countries, as part of a growing commitment to both neoliberalism and social democracy (Cash et al., 2013; Gauld, 2009), economic principles along with individual responsibility rhetoric have been brought in to lower costs (Davis and George, 1993; Bella, 2010; Wyatt et al., 2010). Treating patients outside of high-cost hospital wards and having families provide the bulk of the care in their homes without financial compensation has been deemed more 'cost-effective' (National Cancer Control Initiative, 2003: 47) – as long as the cost of lost income and the health impact of caregiving on carers is not taken into account (Blank and Burau, 2014). 'Hospital at home' (White, 2006: 105) and 'care in the community' have replaced institutions as the location where most medical services are provided (Duckett, 2004: 206).[9] Community services are now the 'glue' (Burns et al., 2004: 501), or quick fix (Petersen, 1994), that allow patients to spend the majority of their infirmity at home. Carers have become the 'backbone' (Kelly and Christou, 2009: 7) or 'central plank of service provision' on which hospital systems depend (Allen, 2000: 150).

Over the past few decades, the demands on family carers have increased (Blank and Burau, 2014). The introduction of economic rationalist practices within hospitals – such as the Prospective Payment System introduced in the USA in 1983 which reduced hospital stays by calculating funding based on the patient's diagnosis and illness at time of admission, regardless of treatment and care eventually given (Bella, 2010) – mean that patients are being sent home 'quicker and sicker' than in decades past (Glenn, 2010: 154). Subsequently, family carers

---

8   Duckett and Willcox (2011: 199), however, suggest that the evidence on the cost-effectiveness of hospital in the home (HITH) is conflicting.

9   Duckett and Willcox (2011: 198–9), while acknowledging that the distinction between the two is not always clear, distinguish between 'hospital-in-the-home' programmes and 'home-based post-acute care'. The former are designed to replace hospital admissions while the latter is designed to promote early discharge from hospitals.

now provide between 60 and 80 per cent of long term care at home (Lewis, 2006; Blank and Burau, 2014; Bruhn and Rebach, 2014d) using complex technology with little training (Bella, 2010).

Political Contexts of Care

Based on the percentages cited above, it is safe to conclude that developed countries now rely on informal caregivers (Olson, 2012). The extent of this reliance, however, and the financial and psychosocial support made available to carers varies dramatically across OECD nations, reflecting a country's 'economic structure, prevailing beliefs, political systems, and cultural practices' (Glenn, 2010: 6). Comparison of the health policies and support offered to informal carers across Sweden, the UK, USA, New Zealand and Australia illustrate the broad range in philosophies and practice.

Sweden has an egalitarian political culture. Taxes are paid in return for a range of entitlements related to minimum living standards, health and social care (Blank and Burau, 2014). Care is cast as a social responsibility in Sweden. Publicly funded health care allows individuals in need of support to remain independent and not reliant on families for this care (Johansson et al., 2011; Blank and Burau, 2014). This is in contrast to countries such as Germany, with more collectivist and family-oriented political cultures, where community interests are prioritised above individual rights or independence. The type of support offered varies across Swedish municipalities, but all offer home help services to patients, including assistance with shopping, cleaning and food preparation (Johansson et al., 2011), reducing a family carer's responsibilities. The Social Services Act also directs municipalities to '"support and provide relief for families who care",' which often takes the form of respite, counselling and financial allowances or reimbursements for carers (quoted in Johansson et al., 2011: 339–40).

Britain, like Sweden, has an egalitarian political culture regarding health, with the National Health Service (NHS) – a universal health care system – being in place since the end of World War II (Blank and Burau, 2014). The strength of this system and the wider political culture in the UK, however, has undergone significant change since the 1980s (Goodhead and McDonald, 2007). A conservative government led by Prime Minister Thatcher, influenced by neoliberal political philosophies, dismantled or weakened many aspects of the UK's welfare state. During this time, the individual and their family were viewed as responsible for providing care to older and disabled citizens. Families who did not or could not provide care were criticised as neglectful (Goodhead and McDonald, 2007). Welfare support was also reduced. Support that was once an entitlement for all citizens was pulled back to merely that of a safety net for only those citizens most in need (Blank and Burau, 2014). Social democratic reforms were (re)introduced in the 1990s (Goodhead and McDonald, 2007; Gauld, 2009). During this time, policies were initiated to promote caregiving as a civic good and to support carers, allowing carers who give care for more than 35 hours a week to become eligible for an Invalid Care Allowance and requiring local health areas to offer needs assessments to carers (Goodhead and McDonald, 2007; Johansson et al., 2011). Compared to Sweden then, the UK is more explicitly reliant on family to provide care, but, in acknowledgement of this reliance, carers across the UK are eligible for social and financial support.

In sharp contrast are the health and social care policies of the USA. The USA is individualistic in its approach to politics: individual freedom is valued above those of the society (Blank and Burau, 2014). Regarding health care, this translates to a largely private medical system where individuals fund their own care through insurance. Medicaid and Medicare were put in place in the 1960s, but these safety net welfare reforms only ensure that those in most need and the elderly are eligible for health care through taxpayer-funded programmes. In the USA the family and not the state is viewed as responsible for care and 'family members (parents, spouses), are [legally] obligated to provide care for other family members' (Glenn, 2010: 9) – especially women. While social programs are available to assist the elderly or disabled citizens with activities of daily living, these social programs are viewed as supplemental rather than an entitlement for all. Unlike Sweden, where there is a concern that reliance on family care will undermine a care receiver's independence, in the USA family are expected to provide care. American policies 'have historically operated on the assumption that the family was responsible for caring for its members and that relatives, particularly spouses, would provide personal assistance gratis' (Glenn, 2010: 107). The current political agendas of carers organisations in the USA revolves around acknowledging each carer's need for support and challenging current policies that disqualify families from receiving public services when there is a family member able to act as a carer (Montgomery and Kosloski, 2014; Kelly and Christou, 2009). Only those most in need, such as a person with a disability without a family carer, are eligible for state support. Legislation was passed in 2010 granting carers of veterans eligibility for training, counselling, respite, medical care and a monthly stipend (Bruhn and Rebach, 2014c), acknowledging the physical and emotional trauma of war on soldiers and the extreme demands this can place on family carers. However, ideological and legal changes will be required before support will be extended to all carers.

New Zealand, while sharing an egalitarian approach to health care with Sweden and Britain, offers little financial support to family carers (Blank and Burau, 2014). As a liberal welfare state, New Zealand introduced their Social Security Act in 1964 (Goodhead and McDonald, 2007). Based in this Act, support, such as home help, is available to patients who are deemed eligible through a needs assessment. Financial benefits, such as the Domestic Purposes Benefit and the Child Disability Allowance, are available to people caring full-time, other than spouses (Goodhead and McDonald, 2007). As of October 2013, New Zealand's Ministry of Health began providing funds to people with disabilities to pay a carer to help with activities of daily living, but spouses of disabled adults and parents of children with a disability are not eligible for these payments (New Zealand Ministry of Health, 2014; Davison, 2013).

The Australian caring context shares similarities with both the USA and UK. Australia's system reflects its British heritage in terms of its commitment to being a welfare state, but has a health care system with a 'strong private component' that reflects some commitment to the individualistic ideals in the USA (Blank and Burau, 2014: 57). Like the UK, Australia introduced a universal health care system called Medibank, though much later than Britain, in the 1970s. Now referred to as Medicare, it means all citizens and permanent residents are eligible for health care through the public hospital system, regardless of income or assets. However, like the USA, Australians are encouraged (through tax incentives) to purchase private health insurance, affording them greater choice in health professionals and shorter waiting lists for elective procedures (Taylor et al., 2008). In terms of policies, Australia has been active in offering support to family caregivers (Blank and Burau, 2014). Like the USA and UK, family are expected to care for sick or disabled family members in Australia. Financial support for carers, however, has been available in Australia since the 1990s through a Carer Allowance and Carer Payment. The former is a modest 'income supplement' for those providing care on a daily basis to a family member living at home with a disability (Blank and Burau, 2014: 218). The latter is an asset-tested payment available to those carers who demonstrate need and/or an inability to work full-time because of their caregiving role. Though Australia has actively acknowledged the important role that carers play through this financial support, in practice, the amounts of support are low, making the Carer Allowance and Carer Payment symbolic recognition for carers rather than full financial support (Blank and Burau, 2014: 218).[10]

The wide range in political ideologies, health care systems and welfare policies that shape contexts of caregiving across developed countries has been aptly categorised by Twigg and Atkin (1994: 13) into four points along a spectrum: 1) 'carers as resources'; 2) 'carers as co-workers'; 3) 'carers as co-clients'; 4) 'superseded carers'. Sweden could be said to occupy categories two to four. While there are attempts to replace or supersede family carers with state-funded human services, in practice many people in need of care prefer to be cared for by their families (Johansson et al., 2011). Thus, most Swedish municipalities offer both psychosocial as well as financial support to families acknowledging their needs as co-clients and co-workers. The USA, in contrast, largely occupies the first category. All but those family carers supporting a veteran are taken for granted as a readily available resource; policies work on the assumption that all persons in need of care have a family member able (financially, physically, technically and emotionally) to provide care without (state-funded) financial compensation or psychosocial support.

---

10   The Carer Allowance, for example, consists of a payment of $118.20 AUD per fortnight (Department of Human Services, 2014). This is a mere nine per cent of the minimum wage in Australia, which is $640.90 AUD per week or $1281.80 AUD per fortnight (Toscano, 2014).

This book examines the lived experiences of carers in one Australian city. Australia can be categorised as occupying categories one, two and three. Carers have been formally recognised since the 1990s as co-workers in Australia through the Carer Allowance and Carer Payment. However, the insufficiency of the financial support and the frequently pronounced calculation that family carers save the Australian health care system billions (Pezzullo et al., 2010),[11] provide evidence that informal carers are also a taken-for-granted resource in Australia. Respite and psychosocial support are available to Australian carers, indicating their treatment as co-clients, but these services are largely outside of the public system, available through employee assistance support, not-for-profit and charitable organisations (Olson, 2012).

While the political and historical contexts of care are important to understanding carers' lived experiences, documenting the various care settings across the globe is not the focus of this book. Past research has established this thoroughly (Fine, 2007; Glenn, 2010; Blank and Burau, 2014; Twigg and Atkin, 1994). The purpose of this book is to examine, from a sociological perspective, and make sense of the varied lived experiences of those informal carers looking after a spouse with cancer.

This book explores the journeys of 32 Australian carers of a spouse with cancer. Cancer is a disease that affects people of every age and can be physically painful for the patient. Once synonymous with death, cancer now follows an uncertain trajectory that vacillates between sickness and health, dying and wellness (McNamara, 2001). This seriousness and uncertainty makes cancer caregiving a form of caregiving distinct from others. For carers of a child with a disability, for example, caregiving responsibilities will likely stretch on for decades. Cancer caregiving, in contrast can last months, years or decades: ending in the cancer patient's remission, survivorship or death; or ending and beginning again with a recurrence. Compared to cancer caregiving, dementia caregiving is often more predictable, characterised by progressive decline in social and cognitive functioning (Meuser and Marwit, 2001). Cancer, however, often eludes prediction. Carers' responses to this uncertainty are a central feature of this book.

Supplemented by other research along the way, this book is based in rich longitudinal interviews conducted with 18 husbands and 14 wives caring for a spouse with cancer in one Australian city.[12] Participants were recruited through snowball sampling and a survey distributed through local cancer and carer support organisations, and a local political party's email newsletter. Participants ranged in age from their 30s to 80s, with most (22) between 50 and 69 years of age. The types of cancer affecting interviewees' spouses ranged from breast (12), prostate (5), neurological (3), haematological (3) and bowel (2) through to rarer cancers

---

11   This report, prepared by Access Economics for Carers Australia, shows that the cost of caregiving is rising, from 30 billion per year in 2005 to 40 billion in 2010.

12   Most participants lived within the city. Others lived in neighbouring regional areas. The spouses of all participants used medical facilities within the city.

(7). Carers were interviewed for the study twice about six months apart, in hospital cafés and other cafés, their homes or a quiet university tutorial room. Most participants (19) were actively providing care to a spouse at the time of our first interview. Others (5) were bereaved carers reflecting on their journeys as carers of a dying spouse or spouses of cancer survivors (8). In interviews, carers were encouraged, over tea or coffee, to tell their stories as they saw it, with prompting limited to what might be considered conversationally appropriate. Following this narrative interview phase, carers were then asked questions about their emotional experiences and use of support services (see Appendices A and B). Each interview was transcribed verbatim and then coded and analysed thematically, to avoid imposing categories on the data and to allow the findings to evolve from continued reading and questioning of the interview data.

In working towards forging a sociological and participant-driven avenue for understanding cancer caregiving, the sociologies of emotion, time and identity as practice are employed to extend our understanding of these carers' experiences further. The resulting 'trail' depicts carers' experiences as: involving new forms of loss and normlessness in time (*temporal anomie*) that are responsive to the way a diagnosis is delivered; varied based on each carer's responsibilities and time sovereignty; and, at times, challenging to one's emotions, emotion work and identity as a spouse. The book concludes by considering the intersections across carers' lived experiences, laying the platform for a sociology of cancer caregiving. It must be noted, however, that this collection and analysis of cancer carers' experiences is by no assessment complete. It is meant to lay a foundation for future practical contributions to cancer caregiving theory, to practice and policy, and to sociology more broadly. Rather than an attempt to 'carve out ... another new specialism' within sociology (Mellor, 1992: 12), this book is an example of the practical and theoretical insights that can be gained from considering cancer caregiving using a sociological lens.

Outline of the Book

Below is a summary of the book, as it is presented in the chapters that follow. Chapters are structured to progress from the immediate changes that a cancer diagnosis can impose on a patient's and carer's taken-for-granted life trajectory to the contradictions and tensions that persist as caregiving continues over months and years.

I begin, following the preface by nurse and sociologist Associate Professor Annemarie Goldstein Jutel, by establishing the relevance of the title 'carer' and by considering what it means to become a cancer carer. Many have investigated cancer patients' illness narratives, from diagnosis through to palliative care or survivorship. For patients, cancer is often associated with the adoption of a patient identity and a statistical probability of death: a 'limbo' between life and death (Halvorson-Boyd and Hunter, 1995). Little and colleagues (1998) refer to this as a persisting sense of liminality. The impact of a cancer diagnosis on a spouse or carer's biography and identity has been the focus of comparatively less research. Recently, there have been calls to abandon the term 'carer' all together, because it is not widely recognised or identified with, and because it is often associated with burden, which has disempowering connotations (Molyneaux et al., 2011). Using Holland et al.'s (1998) identity as practice theory, I present participants' differing reflections on and identification with (or rejection of) the title. Findings depict identification with the 'spouse' and 'carer' label as relationally situated and dependent on meaningful interaction. Participants pose identification as a carer as symbolising a shift in their relationships, from interdependent to dependent. For this reason, some resist and others embrace the term. The label is also used strategically by some spouses, to position themselves as entitled to inclusion and support. Rather than viewing the term as either a failure or a success, I show the label as contextual, positional and enacted, not fixed. I depict resistance to the term as, potentially, a means of symbolically opposing cancer and one's spouse's dependency. I highlight the title's value as an 'artefact' that allows carers to position themselves as entitled to inclusion and support. Thus, in Chapter 1, I ask readers to begin their journey into considering cancer caregiving from a sociological perspective by shifting their thinking about the term: away from questions of the term's acceptance towards analysing what the term's acceptance or rejection can tell us about a carer's experience.

In Chapter 2, I examine carers' diverging stories of loss and grief across carers, prognoses, symptoms and time. Some carers experience the psychological loss of a spouse, when a cancer diagnosis causes their personality and independence to atrophy. This type of loss is associated with anticipatory grief, where the emotional response to the psychological loss occurs a substantial time before the physical death. Other carers' experiences of grief are limited to the physical loss. This happens when an aggressive but asymptomatic cancer goes unnoticed until the patient is diagnosed within the terminal stage. 'Conventional grief' is a typical response to this more sudden form of loss. As survival rates improve, however, cancer journeys more often follow a jagged path based on multiple probabilities. Thus, many carers' experiences are now characterised by uncertainty and oscillating emotions of hope, grief and a desire for normalcy. This prompts what I define as *indefinite loss*: when the extent to which a cancer diagnosis will affect or curtail a patient's life is unclear. This type of loss is characterised by changed priorities, a reduced ability to plan and a more present-focused orientation in time.

Investigating spouse carers' emotional responses to a cancer diagnosis is the focus of Chapter 3. Few have explored carers of cancer patients' emotional journeys, outside of psychology. Within the psycho-oncology literature, some argue that the maladaptive coping strategy denial is prevalent amongst carers. But, using a sociological depiction of carers' emotional responses to cancer, I show denial to be one of many coping strategies used by carers to manage their emotions in the short-term. In the long-term, carers undertake 'emotion work' (Hochschild, 1979; 1983) to actively manage their own emotions towards the future and adapt to a new orientation in time. Carers describe the diagnosis as temporally transformative: disruptive to their taken-for-granted assumptions of a future together with their spouse. For many, this results in a feeling of stasis and normlessness in time, what I refer to as *temporal anomie* (Olson, 2011). The extent to which diagnoses are temporally transformative, however, hinges on the stage, type and predictability of the cancer as well as the way in which the prognosis is delivered.

Although many carers experience the emotions associated with a spouse's cancer diagnosis individually and internally, their emotions are also social: a shared experience with their spouse, family, circle of friends and even culture. Chapter 4 depicts the emotion management that most carers of a spouse with cancer feel obligated to perform with and on their spouse. Drawing again on interactionist emotions sociology theories, primarily Hochschild's (1979; 1983) theories on emotion management, I depict the internal emotional struggle that many carers describe when the time dedicated to caregiving continues and neither death nor cure eventuate. First, I explore descriptions of how a carer 'should' feel – the normative expectations referred to as 'feeling rules'. Second, I describe *spouse* feeling rules. Finally, I show how the vacillating and unpredictable trajectory of many contemporary cancer diagnoses and symptoms causes many spouse carers to feel conflicted about how they should manage their emotions as both spouses and carers. This approach to understanding carers' emotions is an attempt to move the reader's thinking beyond individualistic conceptualisations of emotions within cancer caregiving studies. Conflicting feeling rules also provided one possible explanation for variations in carers' experiences.

In Chapter 5, I describe time sovereignty, based in Goodin and colleagues' (2008) work on discretionary time as a measure of welfare, as another important dimension for unpacking differences in carers' qualitative experiences of caregiving and support service preferences. Quantitative studies based in psychological approaches to understanding caregiving show age and gender to be predictors of variation in cancer carers' experiences, but questions around why this variation persists remain unanswered. During qualitative analysis it became clear that cancer carers' experiences greatly vary depending on how much control carers have over their time. Carers with little to no control over their time, due to juggling multiple roles, lack time to feel. They view emotions as an 'indulgence' they cannot afford. These carers have little time to themselves to sort through their (sometimes conflicted) emotions and little time to enjoy the benefits of caregiving: feeling closer to their partner. Not surprisingly, time destitute carers express preferences for practical support including financial aid and respite. Carers with little to moderate control over their time due to managing one intensive caring role have more time to feel and describe cancer as a source of enhanced closeness with their partner. For spouses retired from paid work caring for a cancer patient with few symptoms, demands on their time are few leaving them an abundance of time to reflect. These carers often seek out support to distract themselves from their emotions or help them in interpreting their emotions. Conceptualising carers' differing emotional experiences based on the amount of control they have over their time illuminates an impetus behind much of the poorly understood variation in cancer carers' experiences and support needs.

The book concludes by proposing a sociology of cancer caregiving to complement the predominantly psychological approaches that have been taken to the subject thus far. The discussion draws together the micro-sociological analyses presented in Chapters 1 through 5, with macro-sociological approaches to improving caregiving contexts. On the whole, the book offers insight into the questions that spouses face when their partners are diagnosed with a life threatening illness: questions around mortality, identity and emotional uncertainty. This insight is extended by an application of micro-sociological theories, which helps us to consider variations in spouses' experiences and to imagine new ways of understanding and supporting carers.

Notes on Terminology

Before progressing, it is necessary to make a few notes about terminology. 'Carer' is used more frequently in Australia and the UK, while 'caregiver' is more often used in the USA. Both terms are used interchangeably in this text to denote the same meaning: a family member providing informal medical, practical and emotional support to a patient. 'Carers of cancer patients' and the less cumbersome title 'cancer carers' are also used interchangeably.

'Emotion' and 'feeling' are two more words used reciprocally in this text. Some distinguish between emotions as the physical and psychological state and feelings as the embodied sensory clues that help a person interpret their emotions (Goldie, 2002).[13] Others, Hochschild (1979), for example, emphasise feelings as learned and controlled states that are worked on to conform to social expectations. I use these two terms correspondently throughout to denote interlinking and inseparable parts of an embodied, personal, social, cultural and interactionist process.

The term 'health care consumer' has been used since the 1960s in place of 'patient' (Irvine, 1996: 192). I, however, use the term 'patient' to denote the person who has been diagnosed with cancer. I do this because it allows for more direct communication and because 'consumer' obscures the unequal power dynamic inherent to the health professional–patient relationship and implies there is a choice in engaging with the medical system, where little choice exists (Irvine,

---

13 Within sociology and cultural studies, theorists such as Massumi (2002) and Hardt (1999) offer yet another category: affect. While interactionist theories dominate the sociology of emotions, the 'affective turn' is gaining traction. Affect is used to conceptualise those sensations and visceral changes that may occur beyond cognition and, potentially, beyond, between and across bodies. It refers to the forces or 'states of being' (Hemmings, 2005: 551) that may go unacknowledged, but nonetheless shape a person's desire and emotion (Poynton and Lee, 2011: 637).

1996). At times, however, the terms 'client' and 'co-client' are used to refer to carers as users of medical and support services who are not the primary users (the patients).

'Health care system' is another commonly used phrase. This system is more aptly referred to by Duckett and Willcox (2011: xvi) as an 'illness care system' because the overall focus is treatment and not prevention. For this reason and because it denotes the biomedical focus to which this system is restricted, this structure will be referred to from here on as the Australian medical system or medical system when referring to the hospitals, practitioners and medical services used most frequently by the participants and their families in this study.

Chapter 1

Identity: Exploring Identity in the 'Figured Worlds' of Cancer Caregiving and Marriage[1]

> What's in a name? That which we call a rose by any other name would smell as sweet ...
>
> Act II, Scene II, *Romeo and Juliet*

Any discussion about names and titles brings to mind the above widely referenced quote from William Shakespeare's ([1597] 1993) *Romeo and Juliet*. It implies the hollowness of titles and their lack of bearing on everyday life – a sentiment that the final scenes of the epic drama and the 'notes on terminology' section in the previous chapter contradict. This chapter explores the importance of the title 'carer' – and identification with or rejection of the title – to spouses of cancer patients' experiences. Starting with an overview of the comparatively well-established importance of cancer diagnoses to patient identities and biographies, in this chapter I engage in the current debate about the merits of the term 'carer'.

Biographical Disruption

Radley (1999: 781) explains that for patients, cancer's biographical impact 'begin[s] at or near diagnosis ... [as] the immediate mobilisation of medical treatment, with its technical vocabulary and its promise of clinical intervention, displaces the everyday world'. While cancer is a biological event occurring within a patient's body, it has profound social, emotional and temporal consequences for patients and their carers. From a biomedical perspective, cancer begins with a 'damaged' or 'imperfect' cell that reproduces, causing a tumour of abnormal cells (Capra, 1982: 389). In a human body with a healthy immune system, these cells are destroyed or quarantined. In a body with a compromised immune system, imperfect cells are allowed to proliferate and spread or metastasise. The effect of these over-reproducing abnormal cells or malignant neoplasms on patients'

---

1 This chapter is a modified and expanded version of the following publication (Olson, 2014a), which has been reused here in accordance with the copyright agreement between the author, Rebecca Olson, and the publisher, John Wiley & Sons Ltd: Olson, R.E. (2014a) Exploring Identity in the 'Figured Worlds' of Cancer Care-Giving and Marriage in Australia. *Health and Social Care in the Community.* http://onlinelibrary.wiley.com/enhanced/doi/10.1111/hsc.12132/.

bodies, identities and biographies is startling, and well known (Remennick, 1998). It begins with the diagnosis.

The diagnosis is the defining moment at which a person experiences 'biographical disruption': an interruption and alteration in a person's life history (Bury, 1982: 167).[2] Hearing a cancer diagnosis from a doctor can change a person's sense of self and future direction. Although this is not the whole of their cancer experience and not the experience of all cancer patients, for many, the label 'cancer patient' becomes dominant (Grbich, 1996: 23), invading all aspects of life and resulting in an 'altered self-image' (Gear and Haney, 1990: 275).

A *cancer* patient identity may be particularly pervasive because cancer, historically, is synonymous with death (Jalland, 2006). As Susan Sontag explains, 'in the popular imagination, cancer equals death' and not just death, but a slow, painful and 'spectacularly wretched' death (1991: 7, 16). Over the past several decades, however, cancer mortality rates have decreased. Cancer is now feared, not because it is certainly connected with death, but because it is uncertainly connected with death. Cancer 'carries the threat of disability and, even more frighteningly, recurrence and the repeated threat of death' (Bard, 1997: 44). Currently, being labelled a cancer patient has a 'secondary consequence' of being persistently seen as possibly, but not certainly, dying (Short et al., 1993: 88).

For those who survive treatment and surgery the journey is not over. Cancer patients whose disease is in remission experience ongoing uncertainty (McNamara, 2000). The probability of a cure hinges on type, stage, surgical and treatment factors. No one is sure if they are cured or doomed and many patients experience ongoing death anxiety (Gear and Haney, 1990; Nathan, 1990; Woof and Nyatanga, 1998). Even after five years of remission (commonly used as a statistical marker of survival) many cancer patients/survivors still feel as though they are living in cancer's 'shadow' (McNamara, 2000: 139), like they are caught between being a patient and person, 'between living a sick role and living a life, and ultimately between life and death' (Frank, 1994: 13).

Often those who are in remission feel as though they are *Dancing in Limbo* (Halvorson-Boyd and Hunter, 1995), between life and death, continually aware of their own temporal limits (Crouch and McKenzie, 2000; Breitbart, 2006). Feelings of abnormality and mortality can persist despite an appearance of recovery and normalcy (Crouch and McKenzie, 2000), because 'cancer narratives refuse to offer the reassurance of complete resolution' (Stacey, 1997: 7). Little and colleagues (1998; 2001) use the term 'liminality' to describe this sense of being between statuses – the heightened feelings of mortality one has as a cancer patient after being on the threshold, but not actually crossing over to the next phase: death. Many survivors remain stuck in this liminal state, between patienthood and personhood.

While patients' experiences of biographical disruption and liminality are well documented, the literature on the experiences of their carers is 'fragmentary

---

2   This is also referred to as 'diagnostic shock' (see Sourkes, 1982; White, 2006: 58).

and diverse' (Thomas and Morris, 2002: 179). Few sociological studies examine carers' experiences of and responses to a cancer diagnosis. Duke (1998: 833) and Grbich (2001: 31), in their studies of bereaved carers, found that families recounted feelings of 'devastation' after hearing the diagnosis. However, the impact of the diagnosis on a carer's biography and identity has remained underexplored. In much of the broader caregiving literature, research findings are atheoretical and focused on burden. There is also a tendency to neglect the diversity in carers' experiences (Greenwood et al., 2009). 'Identity', in particular, is often used without definition or acknowledgement of the concept's complexity. More often, researchers have examined family members' impressions of the term 'carer'.

The Title 'Carer'

Following the changes in the structure and funding of the many medical systems described in the previous chapter, care is now more often carried out within the home by family and friends (Duckett, 2004; Sjolander and Ahlstrom, 2012). Family and friends have been re-labelled 'carers' or 'caregivers', signifying their increased responsibilities as patients move from hospitals to communities. Emerging from the feminist literature, the term 'carer' was introduced to acknowledge the roles and challenges of family or friends who assist a person with a 'disabling condition' at home (Netto, 1998; Blum and Sherman, 2010: 244; Given et al., 2012). The term was also intended to improve the support provided to carers within medical systems and communities (Molyneaux et al., 2011). While policymakers have embraced the term 'carer', some researchers argue that the title is not widely recognised and has disempowering connotations.

Despite the challenges and new activities imposed upon carers, and their subsequent 'lost ... identity' (Mutch, 2010: 214) research indicates that few family members identify as a 'carer' (Aubeeluck and Buchanan, 2006; Williams et al., 2009; Ugalde et al., 2012). Spouses have been described as, potentially, most resistant to identifying as carers. Corden and Hirst (2011: 218) found that this is likely because 'caring for a spouse or partner is widely regarded as an extension of the love and support that define many such partnerships'. Lack of identification as a carer, however, is problematic. Rejecting the title often prevents carers from accessing relevant health and support services, as carers must define themselves as such before seeking out this support (Corden and Hirst, 2011). In a study conducted by the American Association of Retired Persons, the National Family Caregiver Association and the National Alliance for Caregiving, identifying as a carer was found to be the most significant factor in predicting whether a carer participates in support services (Hoffman, 2002). Older spouses suffering from psychological distress are more likely to identify as carers (Corden and Hirst, 2011). A minority of spouses begin to see themselves as parents when their spouses grow dependent upon them to feed, wash and change them (Mutch, 2010).

Molyneaux and colleagues (2011) describe the term 'carer' as a 'universal failure'. While acknowledging that carers' experiences differ depending on the care recipient's illness, Molyneaux and colleagues (2011) have called for the abandonment of the label 'carer'. Based in a convergent review of the literature on carers of people with cancer, dementia, intellectual and physical disabilities and in palliative care, they argue that the term is associated with burden and that most prefer the titles spouse, child, parent or friend. However, in one of the studies included in their review, a telephone survey of over 4,000 Americans, 20 per cent of those who met the criteria identified with the term and 15 per cent did not (Kutner, 2001). In line with Kutner's results, Corden and Hirst (2011) describe both resistance to and identification with the term.

These and other studies point to a need to understand caregiving, and identification as a carer, as more than a success or a failure (Molyneaux et al., 2011), but as something temporally and contextually located. Studies that take a longitudinal approach, for example, are beginning to show changes in carers' overall perceptions and experiences seven months, one year and two years after diagnosis or treatment (Greenwood et al., 2009; Cassidy, 2013). Further qualitative research is needed to understand the processes and circumstances under which caregiving leads to identification as a carer or rejection of the carer identity (Corden and Hirst, 2011; Ugalde et al., 2012).

This chapter takes a participant-driven approach and uses a sociological lens to examine spouse cancer carers' diverging perceptions of the term 'carer'. While many participants describe the cancer diagnosis and new responsibilities associated with treatment and recovery as significant and challenging, few of the spouses interviewed for this study resolutely identified as carers. Instead, participants critiqued the term as devoid of meaning, viewing caregiving as part of their marriage vows. Several, however, qualified their critiques saying they would identify as a carer if the reciprocity in their relationship extinguished. In an attempt to make sense of participants' responses to the title, I then follow suggestions from Ugalde and colleagues (2012) and Thomas and Morris (2002) and draw on interactionist micro-sociological theory to make sense of carers' diverging experiences. Specifically, I use Holland et al.'s (1998) symbolic interactionist conceptualisation of identity as relational, negotiated, situated, and both socially prescribed and individually constructed.

Using Holland and colleagues' socio-cultural 'identity as practice' theory, I depict identification with the 'spouse' and 'carer' label as situated within relationships and dependent on meaningful interaction. When reciprocal practices within the 'figured world' of marriage are maintained, carers identify as spouses. When meaningful interactions diminish, spouses may respond by authoring identities as carers, thus positioning themselves as entitled to support. This portrays identification with the label as contextual, positional and enacted, not fixed. Furthermore, I show that the title 'carer' is not lacking in meaning, but has value, providing carers with an opportunity to position themselves as in need of support, and providing health professionals with a possible indicator of a spouse's increased burden.

Giving Care

When asked to tell their carer story in interviews, participants typically began with their spouse's discovery of a worrying lump, a suspiciously attentive X-ray technician, the shock of the diagnosis or the speed with which their spouse was funnelled towards surgery and treatment. They often recounted the abrupt change in their life direction after hearing '*the* word [cancer]' (Fiona, 60s, spouse with prostate cancer). Participants described their spouses' diagnoses as life course disrupting and their caregiving roles as challenging and encompassing. They described how life was different and what tasks they completed as part of their new carer responsibilities.

For the majority of participants, cancer caregiving meant doing everything possible to prolong their spouse's life on the 'off chance that something in [the patient's] body might switch and might be able to fight' (Marian, 50s, spouse with neurological cancer). This was no small matter. One widower said that caring for his wife was the most challenging job he had done in his life:

> It feels like a huge part of my life ... like a very big item. I have done lots ... high impact and big changes in life, but that's the biggest, ever. And not because it's sad, just because of the power or how overwhelming it is ... It all pales in insignificance when you go through something like that [caregiving]. (Kyle, 40s, spouse with breast cancer)

Prolonging a patient's life entails practical tasks including assisting with mobility and managing medical requirements at home and in the hospital. Tyler (60s, spouse with haematological cancer) described the role as that of the 'case manager' at the hospital. Sally (40s, spouse with bladder cancer) saw it as being the 'organiser' at home, in the hospital and with support services. Kyle assessed that his 'role was to learn how to look after my wife firstly, and then carry that through'. To this end, he kept a 'check on what drugs' she was taking and how much, saying, 'It's ... a bit of an administrator [role] I suppose'. Marian (50s, spouse with neurological cancer) went even further, making charts to analyse her husband's responses to medication and suggest alternatives.

> [My husband] was allergic to the first two drugs of choice for anti-seizures. The third one wasn't working ... it became less effective with time and I had it all documented of when he had seizures, how long they were ... what time of day, and some of these things are fairly time dependent, exercise dependent, food dependent so I had it all on a graph ... and I said, 'look it isn't working and ... what about these drugs?'.

Sharon (50s, spouse with neurological cancer) similarly saw her role as that of the 'advocate' in the hospital:

> I see myself as his advocate … when he is lying in the hospital bed and his feet are sticking over the end and they say, 'the bed is too short' and they say, 'oh I'll get you an end for it' and then they still don't get an extra end. I can go and say … 'Could you?' … So I am the one that does that and gives him the ice to sip and makes sure he has got water and drink. Or if he is not feeling well and vomiting or something I am the one who says look this is happening or that is happening so I am there all the time. And I have made a point of being informed, not to the point of being a pain, but informed to the point of being able to ask sensible questions to know what is going on.

In addition to their new roles as patient and advocate, prescription manager and overall organiser, some carers described their commitment to doing everything possible to prolong their partner's lives as involving research and dietary changes. Marian (50s, spouse with neurological cancer), for example, explained the centrality of organic cooking to her role.

> I looked on my role, initially was to keep [my husband] for as long as possible, to do everything I could to that end. That meant finding out information and then acting on it. Very quickly it became clear to me that organic vegetarian was the way.

These dietary changes, however, could be quite onerous, with Marian describing the hours she regularly spent making hummus from scratch. Anne (30s, spouse with glandular cancer) described her book on nutrition and cancer as her 'bible', reading it every spare chance she had. Based on the recommendations in the book, she altered her family's diet, reducing their intake of meat and increasing their intake of raw vegetables – a similarly time-consuming task that necessitated rising early in the morning.

> R: What kind of role do you see yourself playing?

> Anne: Nutritionist (laughs). That is what he [my husband] calls me. My friends ring up and he is like, 'Would you like to speak to my nutritionist?' (laughs) … I mean we have always eaten pretty well, we just upped it a huge notch … I just took control and it was like right … 'this is what you are going to do'. Didn't have one argument from him, even when he was drinking beetroot juice every day.

> [Later in the interview]

Anne: I would be up at five a.m. in the morning to have to get everything ready and to be able to do it [cooking and organising] to get myself dressed for work and get my daughter to childcare.

Participants also described changed priorities as a consequence of their spouse's cancer diagnosis. In Phyllis's (50s, spouse with neurological cancer) words, 'you [become] focused on looking after the person, making sure all their needs are met' and thus there is little room for the carer's own priorities. Put another way, the patient became the 'prime focus' (Fred, 60s, spouse with melanoma cancer) and 'you come last' (Marian, 50s, spouse with neurological cancer). When I asked Sally (40s, spouse with bladder cancer), what she saw as her biggest needs, she replied, 'I honestly haven't given much thought to what I need at all. I sort of feel that that's way down [in] the priorities'.[3] In addition to changed priorities and new practical and medical responsibilities, the carer role involved fulfilling other family and financial commitments that the patient could no longer manage, such as housework, childcare, earning an income and paying household bills. To complete these tasks and keep the family afloat, many carers managed multiple roles.

Being a caregiver was described as particularly challenging for younger and inexperienced carers. Older carers often had some previous experience with caregiving. Many had cared for a parent in their final years or months, seen more people die and overall had more opportunities to interact with or care for friends or relatives as they were dying. Having had these experiences, the emotional, support service and hospital system challenges inherent to giving care might still be confusing, but they were mysteries that these more experienced carers felt confident in solving.

Those who had not cared for anyone before or had seen few people face death felt ill-prepared for their role. In the absence of relevant experience, some relied on their work experience to guide their actions, prompting one carer to intermittently act like a nurse to her husband, concealing her emotions and shutting out her husband (Millicent, 60s, spouse with haematological cancer). Many said caring required self-education through internet research, seminar attendance and counselling. After caring for his wife through palliation, Kyle (40s, spouse with breast cancer) even said he wished there was a course on 'dealing with dead loved ones at school' saying that 'the two certainties in life are death and taxes' and they do not teach either one in standard secondary school curriculum. Even those who had been carers before found it was a poorly understood role with many reporting uncertainty about their emotions, the ideal degree of hopefulness, their role within the medical system and the support available to them.

---

3 This finding is supported in the literature. Carers tend to prioritise their own needs as second to patients' needs, if they recognise their needs at all (Boulton et al., 2001; Thomas et al., 2002; Morris and Thomas, 2002). Spouse carers, in particular, are the least likely to be concerned with their own health needs (Jansma et al., 2005).

Reflections on the Title 'Carer'

Despite the many challenges, changes to their lives and added responsibilities, few participants strongly identified as carers. Rodney (30s, spouse with breast cancer), for example, said:

> I don't think the role is any different to when [my wife] has been sort of fully fit and healthy. I mean it is that of a husband and father and, but ... there is no doubting it's a life changing experience.

Charlie (50s, spouse with breast cancer) similarly rejected the title, seeing it as nothing 'out of the ordinary'.

> R: What was your role throughout the experience?
>
> Charlie: Well other than just normally being her husband?
>
> [Later on in the interview]
>
> Charlie: I suppose I have been a carer, her sole carer in terms of moral support and providing food and sustenance ... but you do that normally anyway. Didn't think that was anything out of the ordinary, you know?

By our second interview, however, Charlie's wife started using the title. 'I really hadn't considered myself as a carer ... often people say, "Oh what do you do?" and [my wife] will pipe up and say, "He is my carer"'. As Rodney's and Charlie's accounts testify, more often than not, participants resisted identifying as a carer. They did so for several reasons: limitations in the term's meaning, prioritisation of their married identities and the centrality of reciprocity to identification as a spouse.

'Carer' – An Emotionally Limited Title

Several participants described 'carer' as a term that was emotionally limited in scope. Marian, for example, described herself as 'sort of the primary carer'. She was a spouse in her fifties whose husband was diagnosed with a terminal neurological cancer which affected his fine motor skills, but not his cognitive abilities. Marian did not think 'carer' adequately captured what she did for her husband during the final months of his life. When I asked her what would be a more appropriate label she replied, 'I don't know what is'. Mary (50s) was providing care to her husband after a prostate cancer diagnosis with few debilitating symptoms. She saw caregiving as associated with performing physical care tasks, whereas she was mostly supporting her husband emotionally.

It's funny isn't it. I guess I don't see myself playing a caring role until he is more obviously physically sick which is silly because obviously the emotional support is possibly even more important than the physical support.

Millicent's (60s) husband had been diagnosed with a haematological cancer more than 10 years before our first interview. Off and on throughout her journey as a carer, Millicent identified as a nurse or carer as an emotion management strategy.[4] This, she explained, helped her to remain 'cool and calm':

I very much turned to … my role as a nurse on these occasions and I think it helps me manage not to get, I can't say not involved because of course you are involved, but it puts me on a different level if I can be more the nurse and the carer than the wife. I can manage things better that way.

Playing the 'nurse' role involved getting more 'matter of fact' when 'he got a little bit, almost weepy'. Her resolve, however, would diminish in the hospital where 'it was more in my face … I would get upset'. Millicent was, perhaps, able to adopt the nurse/carer role intermittently because of her past profession and because of the changes in their marriage.[5]

Our close relationship has slipped quite a lot in the last few months. There is no sexual side to it anymore …. We are sleeping in separate beds because his bronchitis acts up a lot at night, and I wasn't getting enough sleep …. Acting as a nurse, as I said, is easier for me than acting as a wife …. For a man that was always doing something it's been really hard for him. He isn't even capable of doing – physically his body is thin and weak, so he is just not capable of doing anything and it is really hard for him.

Caregiving as Part of a Marriage

Whereas Marian, Mary and Millicent found (or in Millicent's case, used) the label 'carer', like 'nurse', to be devoid of intimate emotions, Leo objected to the term's bureaucratic origins. Leo (60s) was caring for his wife who had been diagnosed with later stage breast cancer. He saw 'carer' as meaningless and used only for political correctness. He prompted this discussion in our interview saying, 'I hate

---

4   Linda (40s, spouse with bowel cancer) was confused about her role and identity as a carer and the emotional connotations of these identities. Like Millicent, she intermittently identified as a carer. See Chapter 4 for a more in-depth exploration of her carer story.

5   Several other carers (Rodney, Andrew, Ian, Mary, Colleen) also noted the absence of sexual intimacy in their relationships due to their spouse's illness or frailty. None of these carers, however, adopted an emotionally removed 'nurse role' approach to caregiving; they maintained a close emotional relationship with their spouse. This suggests the importance of not just sexual intimacy, but reciprocated interactions and closeness.

the word "clients" which has come to replace patients … it's very obnoxious … . Not calling a spade a spade'. So I asked, "'carers" … What's your impression of the term?' He replied, 'I have some gut reaction against "carers" … the very name irritates me. It's like "significant others", one of those portmanteau words that don't really mean anything and can mean everything'. I asked, 'is "husband" more encapsulating of your role?' He declared, 'You can't improve on husband and wife … it is an act of complete commitment for life … so I don't think it needs to be supplemented by additional role descriptions'.

Leo was not alone in viewing marriage as encompassing of one's carer role. Many, including Rodney and Charlie cited above, described caregiving as an expected part of marriage. Caregiving is 'automatic' (Blake, 40s, spouse with breast cancer). It was seen as the 'in sickness or in health' part of their marital vows. Leo (married 27 years) elaborated, 'we're [a] family, standard, old-fashioned, you know, for life type of marriage and it's just normal … it's just unfortunate that this [cancer] happened to us'. Leo did, however, qualify his statement: 'I think it depends on the quality of the bond between husband and wife'. Carl (70s, spouse with lung cancer), echoed Leo's assessment of the title saying, 'I was a carer, but mostly I saw myself as the husband who took over in times of difficulty', when chemotherapy all but confined his wife to her bed for three months. Andrew (60s), whose wife was diagnosed with breast and gynaecological cancer, described his role in similar terms.

> You don't see yourself as a carer. I mean we have been married in October 40 years. It's something that you think, 'Oh, I guess that's an aspect of it'. But it's just the relationship, who we are, you know, married that long. So I didn't see it as a caring [role]. And when she was first sick … she was in bed a lot and I was doing all the housework and everything. As she has gotten better … we still share quite a bit … . So that's where I'm caring, I mean it's being there, it's part of that relationship, for a long time, but I don't see it as being special. It's just the way we are really.

Fiona and Mark were a couple in their sixties who had taken turns as cancer carers when Fiona was diagnosed and treated for breast cancer and when Mark underwent surgery and long-term recovery for prostate cancer. They described cancer as 'the worst thing that's happened to us in forty-something years'. Nonetheless, because of the long-term nature of their relationship, involving intermittent periods of illness, wellness and care, they viewed caregiving as part of their marriage.

> Well … we've been together for a long time, so I guess we have always more or less looked after each other and this was just another instance, if a little different, with [the] potential to be a bit more serious … . Perhaps it's a life-long partnership thing, but then [it has] been amplified a little bit.

Giving care was seen as part of a marriage: a way of 'returning the favour' to a spouse for times past when roles were reversed. Linda (40s, spouse with bowel cancer) summed this viewpoint up, explaining that caregiving 'is actually about a demonstration about how you feel about that person and how you want to be the one to look after them because you love them'.

Reciprocity

Reciprocity was another impetus behind participants' resistance to identifying with the title 'carer'. Only when physical or psychological changes hindered the emotional and interactive bonds of their relationship would the spouse identity give way. Sharon (50s, spouse with neurological cancer), for example, saw herself and her husband as sharing the carer and spouse roles as part of a reciprocated relationship. When I asked her, 'Who would you say supports you?' she replied:

> It's [my husband] because I will often say to him whatever is happening, 'this bothers me' and 'this worries me', and he is actually very good in some senses to talk to. So although he is the source of the problem, he is actually very good as [both] the supporter [of the carer] and the carer as well.

Judy (60s), who was caring for her husband who had been diagnosed with an asbestos-related cancer three months before our first interview, saw the term 'carer' as somewhat appropriate during our first interview. However, in our second interview she clarified that she identifies as a wife and will continue to do so until her husband can no longer share meaningfully in their interactions. In our initial interview, I asked Judy to start:

> R: From the beginning, when you first saw yourself as–
>
> Judy: –As a carer?
>
> R: If you agree with that word?
>
> Judy: I can't think of an alternative, so we will stick with that .... It's what you do when you get married .... I not only feel I should do it, but I want to do it.

During this interview, she explained that her husband was 'very dependent' and unable to manage his own medications.

> He was not capable of doing anything like administer his drugs or cook his meals. I mean he could wash himself, thank god. And toilet himself .... I do his food. I do his drugs and all his medications.

While Judy agreed with the term to some extent, she saw prescription management and cooking as part of her responsibilities as a wife. During our second interview Judy clarified her appreciation of the term further:

> Judy: I don't really think of myself as a carer. I mean we still have a life. It's not like someone who has got a person [who] really can't give anything back. I mean [my husband] does give back enormously. We still talk about politics. We still laugh at the cartoon in the paper … there is still a lot of giving from him.
>
> R: When do you think you will define yourself as a carer?
>
> Judy: I don't know, when he can't answer me back (laughter). No, I just think I am a wife. I can remember when [my husband] was first quite ill when he came out of hospital and [my daughter] said, 'mum if you need a weekend off … I will come and look after Dad'. I said, 'I don't need to go away love. This is what being married is!' And sometimes when [my husband] is grovelling, grateful for some small thing, I say, 'That is what I am here for'. So I just think it's my job.

Judy said the carer role would remain secondary to her wife role until the point when her husband could no longer respond in conversations, when his disease prevented her from feeling as though she was part of a reciprocated relationship.

Identifying as a Carer

Phyllis's caregiving role began at the point of depleted reciprocity. Phyllis (50s) and her husband were living in a country town when he collapsed one afternoon, becoming ill quite suddenly. They initially thought it might have been a stroke, but they soon learned that her husband had a terminal neurological cancer which, because of the part of the brain affected, had a profound impact on his personality, memory and cognitive functioning. Shortly after the diagnosis, they moved to the city to be closer to medical services and family.

Phyllis strongly identified as a carer. While her experience is unique to this study, it resonates with Judy's long-term assessment that lacking reciprocity is linked to identifying as a carer, and Leo's assessment that it 'depends on the quality' of the relationship. In our first interview, I asked Phyllis how she saw her role while she was caregiving. She replied:

> Really the carer role and the advocate. He had a lot of cognitive problems. In the beginning if you asked him if there was something wrong he would say, 'There was something wrong with my heart'. I would say, 'No, no, no …'. And he would just look at me and he couldn't cope with it …. He would get words wrong and muddled up.

He needed constant care. So I gave up work completely … to mind him full-time. I was just worried leaving him because he would think green disinfectant was green cordial and try and drink it. Or … one day, he'd say, 'What do I do with a toothbrush? I don't know what to do with it'. The next day he could clean his teeth properly, but he wouldn't know how to shave for example …. I don't think he would have been able to use the phone competently if there had been a fire or if he collapsed he would have just waited until I got home.

So that was my main aim, just to make sure that he was cared for and comfortable and got the best treatment possible. Plus I find that in hospital you really have to advocate for the patients. You really have to be there to make sure they get the care [they] need … especially with someone like [my husband] …. There was endless appointments …. That was my role. It was a pretty big role.

Phyllis's caregiving role was demanding, as she could not leave her husband unattended and received only six hours of respite a week. The changes from the cancer to his personality also had a dramatic impact on their relationship:

Phyllis: He wasn't the same, there wasn't a lot of emotional interaction … We were a very close couple so when we went for a walk we would always hold hands wherever we went, and all of a sudden we stopped doing that …. I would do it [hold his hand] and he would just drop it straight away …. So all of that sort of stuff stopped. So that was hard.

R: Kind of a huge – it sounds like breaking up before you …

Phyllis: Yes it is. It's almost like that. When he first got sick I think I cried for about six weeks.

The lack of reciprocity in their relationship exacerbated her sense of burden associated with the demanding nature of the work involved. After their relationship as a couple all but ended, she wanted to be free of her caring role. When MRI scans would come back showing that the tumour had not grown and her husband was going to live in the near future, the doctor presented the news as if it were a relief, but Phyllis did not see it that way.

The real conflict was when he had MRIs and half of you would be saying 'Please', I'd groan, 'Say that it's going to be over soon'. And then the other half of you is thinking, 'Oh that's awful'. And then it would be a while and it [the scan] would come back and it was normal … I would go into a depression for days and I would feel really guilty because there had been no change. And I'd think, 'This could go on for years and I could be locked into this situation'. And people say, 'That's wonderful, isn't it? And I would have to put on this big act and say, 'Oh that's great there's no change. I'm so happy!' I am not a very good actor. This sort of farce would go on, 'cause that's what people expect you to say, and I am thinking, 'If only you knew, this is just a nightmare'. And then of course if there was a change you couldn't say 'Oh it's great, he's got worse! It's all going to be over soon for me'.

As time went on, Phyllis began developing her own health problems. But, she found that her GP was dismissive of her needs. She subsequently sought a new GP who would treat her as both carer[6] and patient: positively reinforcing her work as a carer (and co-worker), and acknowledging and treating her physical and psychosocial distress (as a co-client):

> Phyllis: He [the GP] virtually said the first time, 'I am really sorry there is nothing more I can do for you'. And it was like he was pushing me away .... Instead of saying 'if you need to come back and see me, do'. It was, 'oh there is nothing more I can do for you, but I am really sorry'.

> R: It wasn't just towards [your husband], it was towards you as well?

> Phyllis: Yeah, it was towards me as well. It was like there is nothing more I can do for either of you. But then when I went to the new one [GP] when we moved and he was great. He would say, 'how are you Phyllis? How are you going? You ring me anytime'. I could. I did occasionally .... He was much more ... understanding of ... my emotional needs ... and more supportive.

Understanding Carer and Spouse Identities

Caregiving can be disruptive to a couple's shared life trajectory, requiring spouses to take on added emotional, physical and financial responsibilities, inside and outside of their homes. Despite these changes and accompanying challenges, few 'carers' of a spouse with cancer identify with the term because of its connotations to detached care and bureaucratic convenience, and the encompassing nature of their marriage vows. The emotionally reciprocal context of marriage featured in spouses' evaluations of the term; as long as meaningful interactions were maintained between the spouse with cancer and the spouse providing care, participants saw themselves as primarily spouses. For one participant, a neurological cancer robbed her husband of the capacity for meaningful exchange, prompting a sense of burden, health problems and an unwavering identification with the title 'carer'. Identifying as a carer permitted her access to support services (respite) and treatment as both

---

6   While Blake (40s, spouse with breast cancer) saw his role as that of a loving husband and did not identify with the title 'carer', as Phyllis did, he found that the title resonated with family and health professionals, saying, 'a lot of people seem to respect that role'.

a 'co-worker' and 'co-client' within medical interactions (Thomas and Morris, 2002; Twigg and Atkin, 1994).

Montgomery and Kosloski (2014) have recently formulated a 'caregiver identity theory' to help sociologists and health practitioners to make sense of family members' diverging identities. They depict giving care and adopting a carer identity as a long-term process where 'the caregiver ... engages in a self-appraisal process wherein a judgement is made about the extent of congruence that exists between the individual's behaviour and his or her identity standard' (Montgomery and Kosloski, 2014: 140). At first, the person sees himself or herself as merely doing more tasks as part of their role as a child, spouse, parent or friend. But, over time, the number of tasks grows and the nature of the responsibilities changes to include activities such as bathing and toileting that would not normally be part of their previous relationship. This causes caregiving stress: 'a discrepancy between what a caregiver is doing and what he or she expects to be doing' (Montgomery and Kosloski, 2014: 145). At this point, the previous role and identity become increasingly untenable and the person providing care begins to see him or herself as a carer.

Montgomery and Kosloski's (2014) theory may explain the experiences of family carers of older adults with dementia. Over time, the disease predictably worsens and family carers do more and more for the person with dementia (Meuser and Marwit, 2001). Cancer, however, as established in the previous chapter, is less predictable. Periods of debilitating treatment necessitating intensive and around the clock care work can dissolve with remission, prompting a return to previous roles, responsibilities and relationships.

Holland et al.'s (1998) theory of 'identities as practice' facilitates a more in-depth and – in light of the experiences and reflections presented in this chapter – accurate understanding of cancer carers' diverging perceptions of and identification with the term 'carer'. Building on theories from Bakhtin, Bourdieu, Vygotsky, Mead, Foucault and others, Holland and colleagues (1998) offer an interactionist conceptualisation of identities as a practice. Identities, they argue, are not 'internalized in a sort of faxing process that unproblematically reproduces the collective upon the individual' (Holland et al., 1998: 169); identities are not solely produced by social forces. Nor are they merely produced by individuals, fixed and unchanging across differing contexts, as is popularly espoused in Western neoliberal ideologies (Holland et al., 1998; Hamilton, 2010). Identities are both individual and social projects. They are informed by 'cultural logics' and social positions, but mediated by individuals (Holland et al., 1998: 40). They are not static and bounded, but individually and collectively 'always forming and reforming in relation to historically specific contexts' (Holland et al., 1998: 284).

Their theory of 'practiced identities' is founded on premises of 'figured worlds', 'positionality' and 'authoring' (Holland et al., 1998: 271–2). Figured worlds are the multiple, historical, social and hierarchical contexts we inhabit, situated within power structures that are made and remade everyday through meaningful actions and activities (Holland et al., 1998). Positionality refers to one's entitlement to resources and status within a figured world, which may vary across contexts (Holland et al., 1998). 'Authoring' refers to the imperative of each individual to respond to figured worlds and one's constrained agency in doing so. Worlds, they explain:

> Must be answered – authorship is not a choice – but the form of the answer is not predetermined ... authorship is a matter of orchestration: of arranging the identifiable social discourse/practices that are one's resources ... in order to craft a response in a time and space defined by others' standpoints in activity. (Holland et al., 1998: 272)

Holland et al.'s (1998) theory of identities as practice is used here to understand spouse carers' identities as culturally located and socially positioned, but pliable and open to individual authoring. It is used to view cancer as but one figured world with meanings and positions in which spouse carers operate within or against. Using Holland and colleague's theoretical framework, marriage and cancer can be depicted as two overlapping figured worlds sustained through interactions. Interactions are the messages and actions with meanings that re-affirm (or challenge) a person's identity and position within a figured world. The figured world of a marriage is reproduced through socially and emotionally meaningful interactions between spouses who, in terms of positionality, are both interdependent on one another and independent.

The figured world of cancer, in contrast, is enacted through the diagnosis. This figured world positions one spouse as a patient (dependent) and the other as a carer (depended upon), involved in a relationship of less emotional significance. The carer position is produced through new responsibilities and numerous caregiving activities performed for the patient. The social force of the diagnosis and its corresponding figured world, however, is not automatically internalised. As Holland et al. (1998) articulate, identities are socially *and* individually constructed. Individuals do have some autonomy in how they respond to figured worlds: in how they author their identities and prioritise figured worlds.

Most participants in this study resisted the figured world of cancer, with its connotations of dependence (Fine and Glendinning, 2005; Weicht, 2011), changed priorities and curtailed futures (Olson, 2011; Olson, 2014c), choosing to position themselves as interdependent spouses. This is in line with the broader caregiving literature. Few spouses identify with the term 'carer', more often viewing themselves as husbands and wives performing care-work as part of a mutually dependent marriage (Hoffman, 2002). An older spouse carer in Corden and Hirst's (2011) study, for example, describes the boundaries of caregiving as difficult to perceive. After decades of marriage, where 'partners loved and cared for each other in many different ways; when both were becoming frail it was hard to pinpoint a time when "care-giving" began' (Corden and Hirst, 2011: 224). For participants in this study, the everyday practices of meaningful discourse and emotional interdependence prompted spouses to continue prioritising the figured world of their marriage and author identities as husband and wife. The mutually dependent nature of the figured world of marriage meant caregiving activities often fit with ease within this figured world.

Few participants in this study, however, prioritised the figured world of cancer, identifying as carers. One participant (Millicent), drawing on her professional experience as a nurse, identified as a carer intermittently. This allowed her to quiet her overwhelming emotional response to her husband's terminal prognosis. Another spouse (Phyllis) consistently identified as a carer. Her husband's neurological cancer deprived their marriage of reciprocal emotional interactions, depleting it of actions meaningful to the figured world of a marriage. In this context, Phyllis positioned herself as a carer within the figured world of cancer. This meant Phyllis was literally *entitled* to support as a co-client and co-worker: to respite and inclusion within interactions with health professionals.

This chapter portrays carer identification as complex; shaped by symptoms, activities and interactions; and not fixed, but overlapping and subject to change. Similar conclusions have been made about cancer patients' perceptions of the term 'cancer survivor': identification depends on cultural contexts, prognoses and the importance of the disease to a person's biography (Khan et al., 2012). The findings offered in this chapter have important implications for understanding spouse cancer caregiving relationships and valuing the term 'carer'. First, the title 'carer' should not be judged as either a failure or success (Molyneaux et al., 2011). It should be viewed as a tool, born within the figured word of policymakers, but used by spouses to manage their emotions, and position themselves as in need of support and entitled to inclusion in health care decision-making. Second, heterogeneity in carers' experiences and identification with the term 'carer' should be acknowledged (Greenwood et al., 2009; Broom and Kirby, 2013). Identification with the title may be a consequence of extended contact with the bureaucratic figured world of cancer (Corden and Hirst, 2011). It may also be an indication of changes in a spouse's figured worlds: an indication of reduced emotional interdependence in a marriage and, potentially, increased burden.[7]

Thus, the term 'carer' should not be abandoned. Identification with the term may indicate the extent of a carer's role, burden, changed relationship and need for support. There is still room to improve the visibility of family carers within medical settings (Blum and Sherman, 2010; Given et al., 2006; Sjolander and Ahlstrom, 2012). Abandoning the term 'carer' may serve to undermine progress made towards carers' inclusion in interactions with health professionals in medical and social support settings. Identification with the title may also serve as an important indicator for family, signifying a carer's need for respite.

---

7   Corden and Hirst's (2011) discovery that psychological distress is a statistical predictor of identifying as a carer supports this contention, but further research is needed.

Conclusion

This chapter offers a sociological analysis of spouses of cancer patients' reflections on the title 'carer', based in a thematic analysis of participants' stories. While others describe the term as a failure (Molyneaux et al., 2011), this argument is based in limited conceptions of identity that undervalue the heterogeneity in carers' experiences. Using Holland and colleague's (1998) social theory of 'identity as practice', I show that carers' identification with the term is based in overlapping figured worlds: one of marriage and another of cancer. With the diagnosis, spouses enter the figured world of cancer, which involves new responsibilities, priorities and challenges. However, the figured world of their marriage sustains superiority as long as the reciprocal practices of that figured world are maintained. If they are not, if the illness diminishes the patient's capacity for meaningful interaction in the figured world of their marriage, spouses may respond by authoring a new identity and positioning themselves in a figured world where their status as a carer acknowledges the dependence of their spouse and entitles them to support. Identifying as a spouse cancer carer, then, is largely contingent on the socio-emotional context of interactions between spouses and likely to change over time. This underscores the continued importance of the term 'carer' as a tool for emotion management[8] and recognition, and as a possible indicator of increased burden.

Having established the value of the title 'carer' in this chapter, in the next chapter I examine spouse cancer carers' experiences of loss and grief. Once synonymous with death, cancer is now more often characterised by uncertainty. Chapter 2 explores the impact of this uncertainty on cancer caregiving experiences. Psychological approaches for understanding carers' grief are extended in the next chapter using sociological and participant-driven approaches.

---

8   See Chapter 4 for an exploration of the centrality of these titles, 'spouse' and 'carer', to participants' emotion work.

Chapter 2

Loss: Indefinite Loss: The Experiences of Carers of a Spouse with Cancer[1]

Anne (30s) and I met at a café on a cold winter morning. Two months before our interview, she and her husband had received the devastating news: her husband was diagnosed with an advanced stage cancer of the glands in his head and neck. Despite the time that had passed since the diagnosis, the information was no less upsetting. She cried throughout the hour-long interview, without embarrassment, asking:

> Anne: Am I allowed to cry during this? … I have done so much crying it's not funny.
>
> R: Would you prefer if we move?
>
> Anne: No, I have cried everywhere.

During our second interview, again at a café but in a different part of the city, Anne was more optimistic and hopeful. By then, her husband had survived a disfiguring surgery, chemotherapy and radiotherapy, which left him with only part of his ear on one side of his face. She was eager to close the chapter on cancer in their lives. But, medical professionals could offer no such reassurance, leaving Anne and her family stuck in their current cancer story, unable to progress to the next 'chapter'. She lamented this lack of encouragement saying:

> The thing that they can't tell us that we find really difficult is that they can't say to us that it is okay, that he is in the clear. So, we … go day by day. And they can't tell us that, even with chemo and radio … . So, we don't know the future. We have a little three-and-a-half-year-old girl. It breaks my heart.

Anne's story, and its lack of resolution, demonstrates the impact of the uncertainty of many contemporary cancer diagnoses and prognoses. Cancer trajectories now

---

1   This chapter is a revised and extended version of the following publication (Olson, 2014c), reused here in accordance with the copyright agreement between the author, Rebecca Olson, and the publisher, John Wiley & Sons Ltd: Olson, R.E. (2014c) Indefinite Loss: The Experiences of Carers of a Spouse with Cancer. *European Journal of Cancer Care* 23(4): 553–61. http://onlinelibrary.wiley.com/enhanced/doi/10.1111/ecc.12175/.

follow a jagged path based on multiple treatments and probabilities. Fulton and colleagues (1996: 1349) suggest that, 'as medical technology prolongs life and facilitates the early diagnosis of terminal illness', conceptualisations of loss and anticipatory grief need 'further scrutiny'. As cancer treatments and rates of patient survivorship improve, cancer diagnoses shift from being associated with a certainly imminent death to a potentially limited future. Uncertainty now typifies cancer caregiving. The impact of this uncertainty on cancer survivors has been described as 'liminality': the heightened sense of mortality that cancer survivors experience after being on the threshold of death and continuing to feel uncertain about the future (Little et al., 1998). They also use the term to describe the oscillation cancer patients experience between identification with those who are future-life oriented and those who are future-death oriented.

What impact does this uncertainty have on cancer carers? Research indicates that family carers also feel that their life narratives have been interrupted by the cancer diagnosis (Harden, 2005). Overall, this interruption entails a 'loss of certain future, loss of role within the family and the outside world, concerns about the burden of caring, issues about sexuality [and] loss of financial security' (Woof and Nyatanga, 1998: 77). Spouses are often the family member most upset by cancer because of the change in their roles, increased responsibility and most acutely, '"their fears and shattered dreams"' (Quinn and Herndon, 1989: 46; cited in Nathan, 1990: 222). Few studies, however, have examined carers' experiences of grief in relation to the uncertainty that characterises contemporary cancer diagnoses.

Caregiver Grief

Studies of grief and loss amongst informal carers focus on bereavement following the death of a patient or the anticipatory grief experienced at the end of a patient's life (Burns et al., 2010; Guldin et al., 2012; Kelly et al., 1999; Marwit et al., 2008; Tomarken et al., 2008; Wright et al., 2008). The caregiving literature is dominated by studies on the grief 'symptomatology' of carers of the elderly, people with dementia and palliative care patients (Fulton et al., 1996: 1,352; Lindemann, 1944). Bereavement or conventional grief occurs when the bulk of one's mourning occurs after a person's physical death (Gilliland and Fleming, 1998). Anticipatory grief, in contrast, occurs when the emotions related to loss arise a substantial time before the person stops breathing (Boss, 1999; Fulton et al., 1996).

Originally offered by Lindemann (1944) to describe the experiences of depression, fear of loss and adjustment to life without their spouse experienced by wives whose husbands were at war, the concept of anticipatory grief has since lengthened. It has been reshaped to incorporate the detachment and patterned emotions (shock, denial, guilt, anger, anxiety, acceptance, relief and sorrow) similar to conventional grief that families experience when they know their loved one will die (Duke, 1998; Meuser and Marwit, 2001; Mystakidou et al., 2006;

Sweeting and Gilhooly, 1990; Waldrop, 2007). It has been expanded to refer to losses in the present and future (Rando, 2000). Carers, for example, might mourn the loss of their previous freedom and the hopes they shared with the patient. Patients might mourn their lost future plans and present loss of their mobility, role and sense of wellness. Thus, anticipatory grief has come to refer to multiple phenomena: to mourning that will occur in the future, is occurring, and has already occurred (Al-Gamal and Long, 2010; Frank, 2008; Mystakidou et al., 2006; Rando, 1988; Sweeting and Gilhooly, 1990; Tsilika et al., 2009). Despite the encompassing nature of the phenomena included within the concept, anticipatory grief is described as a 'compelling' concept and is the focus of much research (Sweeting and Gilhooly, 1990: 1,073).

Research on relatives of the very elderly indicates that these carers grieve anticipatorily because the older person goes through a social death before their physical death (Gilhooly et al., 1994). Patients become increasingly dependent on others for pain medication and mobility (Nash, 1980). Dependency on others may result in a shameful and 'spoiled identity' (Goffman, 1968) and a slow loss of dignity: a loss of 'those characteristics of a person and the environment which allow [them] to feel an identity, a sense of self worth, a sense of stature' (Nash, 1980: 65). Consequently, the elderly can suffer a loss of value to their family and wider community and exclusion from family decisions and community events. Their decline in status, inclusion and dignity results in a tacit and unofficial social death (Elias, 1985; Pine, 1980). The family and carers of the elderly tend to mourn this social death, or loss of the person they knew, and adjust to a life without them well before the patient's physical death. Thus, family often experience the bulk of the physical and psychosocial responses to their loss – the anxiety, depression, sleep disturbance, digestive trouble, loneliness and sense of meaninglessness – while the person is still alive (Neimeyer et al., 2002; Fulton and Fulton, 1980; Gilliland and Fleming, 1998).

Dementia carers grieve anticipatorily, for similar reasons. As their family member grows less lucid, they mourn the loss of the social person with whom they had a relationship (mother, father, spouse) as well as the future 'bodily death' (Meuser and Marwit, 2001: 659). Braithwaite, for example, found that the loss of the social person was cause for anticipatory grief amongst dementia carers. Watching the dementia patient's 'intellect and personality degenerate' was statistically related to 'minor psychiatric symptoms in carers' while physical deterioration was not (Braithwaite, 1990: 77). These carers detach from their relationship, but not without guilt. As Meuser and Marwit (2001) explain, based in their research into the stages of grief of dementia carers, carers continue to care emotionally and physically for the patient, but often under a redefined relationship where the carer views him or herself as the parent and the patient as the child. Carers of a parent with dementia often grieve for the lifestyle they have lost after taking on the many responsibilities associated with caregiving. Carers of a spouse with dementia often grieve for their lost relationship. The death of the person with dementia is experienced as both a relief and cause for further mourning (Meuser and Marwit, 2001; Gilhooly et al., 1994; Gilliland and Fleming, 1998).

Child development and family studies expert Pauline Boss (1999) refers to this mismatch between the physical and social death of a loved one as *ambiguous loss*. As Boss (1999: 6) explains, 'people hunger for certainty'. With ambiguous loss, however, the loss is anything but certain. It occurs in two types. In one, the lost person is 'physically absent but psychologically present, because it's unclear whether they are dead or alive' (Boss, 1999: 8). A person who has gone missing is an example of this first type of ambiguous loss. Typically the family have difficulty in moving forward and creating a life without the missing person because it is not clear if or when they will return. In the other setting, 'a person is perceived as physically present but psychologically absent' (Boss, 1999: 9). A family member who has Alzheimer's disease is an example of this second type of ambiguous loss, which leads to anticipatory grief.

Those experiencing ambiguous loss typically feel very alone in their mourning. There is no funeral or other religious or community ceremony to mark the loss (Boss, 1999). As a result, 'their experience remains unverified by the community around them, so that there is little validation of what they are experiencing and feeling' (Boss, 1999: 8). Those feelings typically consist of mixed emotions and thoughts. Families experiencing ambiguous loss typically feel both anger towards their loved one for 'keeping them in limbo' and guilt for feeling angry (Boss, 1999: 61; Gilliland and Fleming, 1998). A person experiencing ambiguous loss might simultaneously 'cling' to and push away their loved one (Boss, 1999: 63). This uncertainty and the lack of finality makes it difficult for people to move on, to restructure 'the roles and rules of their relationship with the loved one' and restructure the direction in their lives (Boss, 1999: 7).

Carers and family of palliative care patients are said to grieve anticipatorily as well, but to a lesser extent. As these patients are more often lucid, families do not grieve the social or psychological loss before the physical death. More often, patients and families offer 'mutual support' to each other (Meuser and Marwit, 2001: 659) and share in emotions with the dying patient (Fulton et al., 1996; Sweeting and Gilhooly, 1990), in addition to experiencing conventional grief after the person's death.

While many studies have examined carers' experiences of grief after a cancer patient's death or immediately before death, in the terminal stage, there is a paucity of research on informal cancer carers' experiences of loss and grief at other points in the, now less predictable, cancer journey. Cancer might have been a metaphor for death in the past (Sontag, 1991), but as the mortality rates for many cancers decrease in Australia, and elsewhere, and survivorship increases, cancer is no longer a death sentence (Freak-Poli et al., 2007). Many cancer illness trajectories now follow a wandering path, with patients' futures based on multiple probabilities and uncertainties (Little, 1995). There is a need to better understand carers' emotional experiences at different stages of their caregiving 'careers' (Frank, 2008: 525).

In this chapter, I explore the loss and grief experienced by spouse cancer carers at various stages of their caregiving journeys, engaging with both the psychological and sociological literature on loss and grief. In addition to conventional and anticipatory grief, analysis of carers' stories suggests that many carers experience indefinite loss. This form of loss characterised the experiences of spouses caregiving outside of the terminal stage. They experienced the current loss of a taken-for-granted certain future, but the future loss of their spouse remained uncertain. Spouse cancer carers described a heightened awareness of mortality, and an inability to plan for the future. Uncertain prospective losses are largely neglected within the grief literature. In this chapter, I offer insight, based in inductive analysis, into the distinct experiences associated with a potential future (indefinite) loss of a partner and offer the concept indefinite loss to extend our understanding of cancer carer loss.

The differences in Phyllis's, Marian's and Linda's experiences illustrate the contrasts in carers' experiences and highlight the distinction between anticipatory grief, conventional grief and indefinite loss. Phyllis, a carer whose spouse's personality changed due to a neurological cancer, experienced anticipatory grief. She mourned the loss of her relationship, her freedom and the future physical loss of her husband. Marian, a carer who worked with her husband to believe they could beat cancer experienced conventional grief, where the bulk of her mourning occurred after her husband's physical death. In contrast, when patients' prognoses were less certain, when they were diagnosed with a life-threatening and not a terminal cancer, carers experienced indefinite loss. While they experienced some anticipatory grief for the present loss of their taken-for-granted plans, the social and physical loss of their spouse had not occurred and it was unclear if and when it would. Linda's story epitomises indefinite loss, which is the primary focus of this chapter. Her experience represents a type of loss articulated by most (26) of the participants in this study.

Phyllis

Phyllis (50s), a carer introduced in the previous chapter, had a distinct caregiving experience. Her husband became suddenly ill as consequence of a terminal neurological cancer. The effect was immediate. He became confused and fixated. He was forgetful and Phyllis had to provide ongoing guidance. His personality also changed. He withdrew, virtually ending their married relationship. For Phyllis, grieving began the day her husband withdrew. After their relationship as a couple ended, she wanted to be free of her caring role; she wanted him to die so it would be over.

> Caring when you know someone is going to die: at some stages you just wish [it] would hurry up and happen because you are so distressed by it all and it's so horrible to watch someone deteriorate like that, to lose someone who has had a really good memory and a really good mind. To watch them get worse and worse

is really horrible. So you end up feeling really guilty because you are wishing sometimes that it would just happen which is awful but, I know other people have said the same thing when you get to the stage where you think, 'oh I just wish this was over'.

As this is a socially unacceptable sentiment, however, Phyllis felt guilt about her feelings. Later on, Phyllis elaborated:

> You just think, 'I wish it would be over'. But, you feel really guilty, because you didn't want it to be over but you wanted to be out of the situation and you didn't want them to be sick.

When her husband did die, it was a relief. By our second interview it had been a year and a half since his death. She had moved on and was settling into a new relationship, because, as Phyllis explained, she began grieving the loss of her husband the day his personality changed.

> I went through a lot of anticipatory grief because I knew he was going to die and he wasn't the same person anymore. So that made it a lot easier for me when he did die because I had already been through all this, I had separated emotionally.

Phyllis mourned the loss of her husband when his personality changed, well before his physical death.

Marian

Marian's experience of grief was quite different. Although Marian's husband also had a neurological cancer, his personality did not change. She spent her caring days wishing and believing her husband would live as part of their complementary medicine approach: doing everything possible, from organic hummus to dried herbs, on the 'off chance' that it would help him and his immune system:

> You can either go down the Western medical model, or you can combine it with the more holistic, some people say Eastern, some people say complementary, approach. There is lots of literature … that says if you give somebody a diagnosis [prognosis], that's when they will die. [My husband], I remember the day perfectly well. A group of doctors, nurses, us, and they said, 'It's bad news. It's six to nine months and virtually nobody lives past … a year … '. [My husband] just looked at them and said … 'I know that's just based on a group of people and I am not average, so I will not listen to you'. He … said that afterwards.

For me it was difficult. I mean my background was in Science … but the other part of you … goes down the [complementary path] … . If you go down that path you have to truly belief that you can beat it.

Our first interview was on the one year anniversary of her husband's death.[2] Marian said she was going to see a grief counsellor because she was still working through her grief. She explained to me on our second interview that she was still grieving for her loss, making time and space to experience her emotions:

I need to make more time for me just to feel … . [I am] trying to work out ways of me slowing down, not rushing around doing things but making time for myself, so I can just feel … I haven't yet [fully felt] the pain of the sadness, which to me is an ongoing thing. There is not an end to that, feeling the pain of the sadness. Yes, and I am not doing that. I will get sad and I will say, come along, get up and do something … . I [now] try not to do much. I try just to say well I will just sit and go and look at the lake and have a cup of coffee. I think the jargon is sitting with the grief (laughs).

Marian's grief followed the more conventional pattern for a widow (Gilliland and Fleming, 1998). Because of their shared commitment to believe that they could 'beat it' her grief was delayed. It followed the death of her husband and was an 'ordinary loss … codified by official verification – a death certificate, a funeral ceremony, and a ritualized burial' (Boss, 1999: 9). It began with physical death, though it did progress along a non-linear course that required her focused efforts.

Linda

Linda's pattern of grief fell somewhere in between Marian's and Phyllis's. Linda's (40s) husband was given a terminal prognosis following a bowel cancer diagnosis. Two years after radical surgery, however, he was living well despite the oncologist's first prediction. The surgery involved a multiple-day-long procedure where the surgeon:

Opens you up completely from neck down to pelvis … removes all the cancer. They cool your body dramatically down, pack you in ice and they soak your insides. They fill a basin with heated chemotherapy, 40 degrees Centigrade and then soak you in it for two hours. Then they drain all that out and they put you all back together and then over the next five days you have tubes that are in you and you get more chemotherapy put in, cold chemotherapy. They are soaked in that for 23 hours and you are turned during that time to [ensure it] makes it

---

2   It is important to note that one year following a loss can be a significant bereavement event. The date of our interview was chosen by the participant and the participant had an appointment with a bereavement counsellor later that same day.

round your body and then they pump it out. And then after that you just go into convalescence.

The surgery is extremely risky, as this quote suggests, and rarely performed, but it meant that Linda's husband went from a terminal prognosis and palliative care to an improved chance of surviving five years.

Linda described her husband's cancer diagnosis as a series of transformations: a terminal prognosis, new hope in the radical surgery and ongoing uncertainty about their future.

> They said there wasn't any hope, that he had sort of months to live rather than years and that he could undergo more treatment for keeping him comfortable but that's all that could be offered. And then we were referred to a guy in [city] … who is doing a very new and controversial treatment. And that treatment has led to my husband actually still being alive today. He is still classed as terminally ill because it is not expected to be a cure …. Most people who have this treatment … three had survived past four years … seventeen had died in years two to three. And we are in the middle of year two.

Going from a terminal prognosis, through a high risk surgery, to a 15 per cent chance of surviving five years drastically altered Linda's expectations about the future with her husband. Instead of planning for his funeral or a long term future together, they were 'liv[ing] for the now'.

> We are on bonus time and we just enjoy that …. The way we look at it, well I don't know if I am going to be here next year either, and I would like to meet a person who can guarantee they are going to be around next year. I don't think that's true of anybody, so we don't worry about that.

The future was too painful to consider and too uncertain. Thus, Linda was both grieving their lost future together and trying not to focus on the future, because the loss was not certain.

Her experiences shortly after returning to work exemplify the uncertainty of her grief. She talked about being unable to plan for the future. She explained that during an exercise at a planning meeting at work:

> The facilitator did this first exercise and she said 'well let's do your personal life first and here is a sheet and I would like you to fill in what you think your goals will be for the next year, for the next three years, for the next five years, and also write down what you think will be happening then'. Now that was too painful for me because I had stopped looking ahead. I was too busy enjoying the here and now and for someone to say to me what will your life look like in three years' time was something I didn't want to think about.

During our second interview she described their sense of precariousness about the future as ongoing.

> The more time goes on, the more you are worried about a huge fall … . Although you are taking it step by step, so a daily approach … I know statistically things aren't good, but I am not going to worry about the numbers too much because nobody knows in this life. I might not be alive next week. So in terms of talking about a prognosis, well we are all going to die one day. I could go before my husband … which hopefully won't happen and of course his risk is much higher, but at the same time, just in living, it's a risk, so I don't dwell on it … . You live more normally in that three month block before the week before his next test when it all comes screaming back to you about, this is so fragile and it might be back and if he is a little bit unwell or something. It's the first thing you think of. You think, 'oh, it might be back!'

During the same interview, she described her financial planning as conflicted. If she thinks about financial plans that exclude her husband she asks herself, 'Why am I having these thoughts? It's almost like saying here is your hat, what is your hurry?' The potentiality of the loss prompted a sense of stasis: an internal back and forth between making future plans and not planning, but living in the present.

The contrasts between Phyllis's, Marian's and Linda's experiences of loss were substantial. Marian's grief could be described as conventional. During the bulk of her husband's illness she believed he would survive. Over his final weeks, however, after he decided to accept no further treatment, they shared an awareness and emotional response to the impending loss. Phyllis's loss was ambiguous and her grief was anticipatory. She mourned the loss of their marriage and her husband's psychological death before she mourned his physical death. Although perhaps not evident to her family or friends, to Phyllis, there was a clear loss before her husband died. She had lost a reciprocated loving relationship and she knew that neither her marriage nor his personality were going to return because the tumour was inoperable. She knew her husband was not going to be part of her future because he had been given a definite terminal prognosis and limited future. At his funeral, instead of devastation, her husband's death was a relief. It was a 'liberating loss' (Elison and McGonigle, 2003): an alignment of the social and physical death; a matching of the person's social death with their biological death.

In sum, 'conventional grief' resonates with Marian's experience, and, by the follow-up interview, the experience of five other carers whose spouses died before our first or follow-up interviews. 'Anticipatory grief' resonates with Phyllis's experience. However, these concepts do not fit Linda's experience. Unlike Phyllis's loss, Linda's had not yet occurred and it was unclear if and when it would. These two aspects of her loss, that it had not yet occurred (physically or socially) and that it was uncertain, represent the distinct nature of cancer carer loss (outside of the terminal stage). Cancer carers outside of the terminal stage, like Linda – which comprised 26 of the 32 participants in this study – were unsure of how to anticipate the future and so they experienced indefinite loss. They grieved for their lost assumptions about the future, for their potentially lost future plans with their spouse and struggled to orient themselves towards a future that potentially, but not certainly, did not include their spouse.

Indefinite Loss

Uncertainty was both a characteristic of the loss and a cause for mourning. Cancer prognoses are associated with statistics to do with the cancer type and stage and the type and success of surgery and other treatment. Thus, the future is based on multiple probabilities and uncertainties. The illness trajectory for cancer follows an erratic path that can vary between periods of extreme illness and relative wellness. However, periods of wellness are not necessarily indications of likely longevity; nor are periods of severe illness during chemotherapy indications of the brevity of a patient's future. So, neither statistical nor observed indicators provide reliable assurance about the future. This ambiguity shapes carers' sense of loss. Decisions had to be based on limited information and, consequently, planning was limited to the near future, leaving carers feeling immobilised in their life course.

For the family of patients in palliative care, the future is certain: death in a matter of days, weeks or possibly months. With that certainty, the family can begin to prepare themselves for the changes they will face and the loss of a close relationship. They begin to grieve anticipatorily. For carers of Alzheimer's and dementia sufferers, the future is also more certain. Initially, some carers, adult-child carers more than spouse carers, question the diagnosis and, over the course of the disease, the patient may share rare moments of lucidity with the carer. However, after the dementia sufferer's symptoms become moderate, the illness trajectory is certain (Meuser and Marwit, 2001). For how long may be hazy, but it becomes clear that the patient will continue to experience decreasing cognitive function and increasing dependence. Consequently, their 'grief escalates linearly' (Meuser and Marwit, 2001: 665). Alzheimer's carers often see their caring career as akin to walking down a series of steps, with each step representing a crisis in the patient's mental and physical health and the final step being their spouse's death (Boss, 1999).

Cancer carers in this study, other than Phyllis, did not experience anticipatory grief, watching as the patient slowly and predictably declined: losing dignity, mobility, bodily control and social identity. For the other carers in this study, illness trajectories were less predictable. Millicent (60s), who had been caring intermittently for her husband with a haematological cancer for 12 years at the time of our first interview, confessed, 'Neither of us knows how far down the track he is towards death ... I don't know how he will go. Nor does he and the doctor's haven't really said'. The diagnosis was clear, but the future was not. The physical loss was not impending or certain; the loss of the social person had not yet occurred. When or if (the patient might outlive the carer) she would lose the physical and social person was uncertain.[3]

Prognostic information was often vague and of little help. Blake (40s), for example, asked the doctor diagnosing his wife's breast cancer, '"Is she going to die?" And he [the doctor] said, "well, everyone dies" … . He said, "She will need a lot of support"'.[4] Even a clearly delivered terminal prognosis was no guarantee of certainty or predictability. Several patients, who had been categorised as terminal initially and given only months to live, were still alive two or even five years later. For example, five years after receiving a six month prognosis, Jane (60s), who was both a cancer patient and a carer, participated in this study as a carer for her husband following his treatment for prostate cancer.

Even after remission, uncertainty continued. Ian (50s, spouse with breast cancer), who was introduced at the beginning of the book, explained, 'It's been over ten years now but, you know, one problem is that … [my wife] is aware that with breast cancer there is a residual chance of it reoccurring'. Only when patients entered hospice care or began displaying clearer signs that death was approaching (such as acute difficulty breathing, extreme weight loss, jaundice or going into a coma)[5] did cancer carers begin to feel certain of their spouse's immediately limited future and thus begin to mourn and plan with certainty for a life without their spouse. Until then, carers experienced indefinite loss. This indefinite loss was characterised by an acute awareness of mortality, a sense that planning, travel and quality of life were limited, the replacement of old priorities with new ones and grief for past laid plans.

Awareness of Mortality

Many carers alluded to being more keenly aware of the finite nature of life. They talked about cancer as 'a cloud of metastatic possibilities hanging over' them, representing their partner's and their own awareness of their indefinite futures (Sally, 40s, spouse with bladder cancer). Leo (60s, spouse with breast cancer), for example, described his wife's symptoms as a constant reminder of his fear.

---

3   By our second interview, her husband had died and Millicent was experiencing conventional grief.

4   This lack of clarity in the prognosis delivery may be because medical professionals find it difficult to engage in conversations on death and the consequently poor quality or contradictory nature of this communication exacerbates this uncertainty (McNamara, 2001; 2000; McNamara and Rosenwax, 2007; Salander and Moynihan, 2010).

5   Blake (40s, spouse with breast cancer), for example, described his wife's state in the weeks before her death, saying, she 'was just increasingly more in bed and less energy … very sleepy and increasingly jaundiced … . She looked [like] she was going to die. That look that people get … very gaunt and body … kind of greyish look. And you know they are not going to make it'.

> A friend of ours died yesterday of cancer. She only had it [cancer] three years
> .... I live in fear with a lump in my stomach. Each time she [my wife] has
> something, you know, an ache, [a] pain, this or that, gets short of breath, I think
> *Ugh* .... So there is a great fear. But ... I am grateful for what we have.

Later on in our interview Leo, who was also a medical doctor, described 'an incident' where he overreacted to a lump, illustrating the extent to which his fears about his wife's future had affected him.

> Often ... in mastectomies ... there is contraction of the tendons and you have to
> do a lot exercises and so on. But there was one that contracted to such an extent
> that it felt like a stone lump and the nurse shouted from the bedroom where she
> was doing the dressing to come [in]. And she said, 'Leo ... come and feel the
> lump'. And I felt the lump and well five minutes later fainted thinking this must
> be the cancer .... I fainted, then got up had a glass of vodka and a smoke and
> recovered then ... the surgeon and he laughed and he said, 'it often happens like
> that. You just have to massage it'. And indeed it wasn't a recurrence.

Carl (70s, spouse with lung cancer) spoke about mortality saying, 'you can see it [death] sort of looming'. Despite ongoing treatment and the continuous improvement being made in cancer therapy, Carl was very aware that statistics for lung cancer were not in their favour. He knew that he would soon have to plan a life that did not include his wife, but when was not yet clear. Andrew (60s) said cancer is 'there all the time ... as soon as you wake up ... then the realisation hits you almost every morning': the realisation that his wife had metastatic breast cancer and, very probably, a limited future. He went on, explaining, 'I mean you know that but when things all of a sudden, it's a hit and that – there is a finite time for [my wife]'. Anne's (30s, spouse with glandular cancer) anecdote provides some comic relief, but also shows the primacy of cancer and mortality in her thoughts. She and her husband became very worried about a lump that was growing more evident above his collarbone.

> He had this lump growing here at the base of his ... throat. And I had been sitting
> across from him having breakfast or dinner, and I was looking at this thing and
> ... I finally said to him, 'you have got a lump on your throat'. He said, 'Yeah, I
> am a bit scared. I have been watching it now for a while. I noticed it about two
> weeks ago'. ... He waited for his next check-up and he finally went and he said,
> 'What about this lump? We have been panicking about it' ... It is very difficult
> the minute you see a change not to think, 'Shit, it's back!' It hangs over your
> head even if you are trying not to let it .... And he [the doctor] goes, 'It is your
> Adam's apple!" .... He has lost so much weight that he has actually got an
> Adam's apple .... And we couldn't stop laughing. We were laughing for days
> about that one.

Fred's (60s, spouse with melanoma) wife Jane, introduced earlier in this chapter, was given six months to live five years ago. Despite her relative wellness, he still worries when she gets headaches. 'It's the uncertainty. It niggles. It depends also on my state of mind too. If I want something to worry about for whatever reason, that springs to mind!' Jane (60s, spouse with prostate cancer), Fred's wife, is also reminded daily of her husband's mortality.

> There is not a day that doesn't go past that I think about dying and Fred. I think about him, every day, about how easy it would have been for him to just die. And I don't dwell on it, but it's a fleeting thought that comes in. I don't know if that will ever stop. It's just something that is there. You just live with it, every day.

Carlie (50s, spouse with oral cancer) explained that, as a couple, their fears about the future were not likely to resolve in the near future because of the probability of recurrence.

> If he gets a headache or his leg aches … he thinks, 'maybe the tumour, maybe I am getting cancer somewhere else', because they say you can get secondary cancer. So that is always going to be in the back of our minds, if it's going to recur.

After more than a decade of caregiving, Sharon (50s, spouse with neurological cancer) described her awareness of mortality and uncertainty as persistent, but easier to deal with.

> So as the time goes on I am getting better at dealing with the fact that we now live with this sort of unresolved set of tumours that are there. But I still keep an eye on him and I am aware of him coughing and just how he is generally. Yeah, so it's always in the back of my mind. It never sort of goes away and I haven't ever forgotten.

Incapacitated Planning

In addition to a heightened awareness of their own and their spouses' mortality, spouse cancer carers experiencing indefinite loss described future planning as limited. Andrew (60s, spouse with breast cancer) said, 'you can't plan too well'. Charlie (50s, spouse with metastatic breast cancer), who I interviewed in August, described planning as limited to seven days in our first interview:

> I … don't plan beyond about next week these days. There is no point anymore …. We don't make any long-term plans. If you said to me, 'What are we going to do for Christmas?' I would say, 'Hang on. That is too far away, wouldn't think about it'.

But, by our second interview his wife's condition had worsened and so had their capacity to plan. 'The future has got down to what I am doing this afternoon almost. Never mind next week stuff'. This prompted Charlie to:

> Live for the moment. Never mind worrying about 20 years down the track. Live for now. You can worry about 20 years down the track when you are 25, but when you are in your 50s – oh bugger it! Live for now! Go and enjoy it.

Rodney's (30s, spouse with breast cancer) experience provides another example. During our first interview he talked about being a 'chronic planner' and making financial plans that excluded his wife. He said, 'I found in making sort of investment decisions, well hang on we can't really rely on [my wife's] income and then feeling guilty for even thinking that', as if he was wishing her away in his planning. Although he tried to make plans, he could no longer do so with a sense of certainty and without guilt. Many other carers reported similar feelings in making important decisions such as purchasing a car or buying a house. This inability to plan for the future and the emotional response when they tried meant that many carers felt paralysed in time. They could neither move forward nor return to a pre-cancer life with their spouse.[6]

New Priorities

A change of priorities was another response to indefinite loss. Sharon (50s, spouse with neurological cancer) noticed a change in how she approached family arguments. Instead of addressing their concerns directly, when her children squabbled she would yell, 'Look for goodness sake; there are more important things in this world. Your father has got a life-threatening disease. Just, stop arguing about who has the last Tim Tam [chocolate biscuit]!' Charlie (50s, spouse with breast cancer) noticed a change in what he worried about and his tolerance for people who worry about 'the small things'. Because of his wife's cancer, Charlie only concerned himself with 'the big picture': health, life and milestones. 'I probably got like that, all these people worrying about other things – go away. Go and worry about something real!' Sally, (40s, spouse with bladder cancer) noted that after she became acutely aware of her husband's mortality, she too reassessed what was important.

> In terms of time, there is maybe another facet to it, which is about reassessing what is important to you when everything – [when] lives flash before your eyes in a short period of time.

---

6   Meuser and Marwit (2001: 266) found that many carers of spouses with dementia also say they can no longer 'look backward' or 'forward'.

Kyle (40s, spouse with breast cancer) summed this up by describing cancer as having rearranged his life priorities: 'it all just jumps up in the air and a few smaller pieces land'.

Mourning for a Taken-for-Granted Future

These carers also talked about mourning their previous plans for the future: their displaced 'dreams, wishes and fancies' and previous plans for the future (Radley, 1999: 781). In couples where the cancer had a debilitating impact, doctor's appointments and ill-health got in the way of achieving the plans that couples had made for their future. Charlie's (50s) wife's breast cancer metastasized to her brain causing her to feel constantly nauseated and necessitating ongoing radiotherapy which limited their ability to travel. Charlie said 'the biggest disappointment', as a result, was not accomplishing 'the hope [from] a few years back that at this time we would be out and about all the time, care-free' enjoying retirement. During our first interview, he lamented their inability to travel outside the city because his wife would need to be close to her oncologist in an emergency or because of their need to attend regular medical appointments.

> At the moment, we sort of live in three-week blocks, because she has to have treatment every three weeks and that will go on until March. I think the normal regime would be two years of that treatment ... . Yeah, it has probably put a big hole in the long-term plans, changed our entire outlook on life.

Andrew (60s, spouse with breast cancer) and his wife similarly found their capacity to travel curtailed because of her symptoms and therapy.

> She finds travelling a little bit difficult ... . We were going to go to Alice Springs. It was going to be a nice big treat for us, but in the end ... she was nearly there ... we did do a three hour drive and she found that a little bit difficult so ... in the end she decided not to do that.
>
> [Later on in the interview]
>
> Every three weeks you've got a chemo [appointment]. Then there is oncology, and then there is the gynaecology. Then there is gastroenterology.

In our second interview, Andrew concluded, 'things you would like to be doing, you don't do'. Ian (50s, spouse with breast cancer), illustrating his grief for their lost retirement plans, went as far as to say:

> There is no point saving money during your life, when you don't know why. You would like to think why you're saving it – you are saving it for a fantastic

retirement. Well, the first thing, it's the realisation more than anything else: that's what we are not going to have together.

Frank (70s, spouse with haematological cancer) also described the importance of living near to a hospital as well as a sense of sadness and frustration at not being able to realise his retirement dreams. He said, 'I am sure most of us think "oh well, when I am 60 and when I get away from work we will have a caravan and travel around Australia"'. But, cancer:

> Changes your life completely, the things that you planned as a younger person, that you were going to [do when you] retire. You were going to go around the world, around Australia .... It doesn't happen anymore. It is just all cancelled. And you just live from week to week.

In an email to me following our interview he wrote, 'Personally, I envy every retired couple that I see on the road in their caravan. I do hope that they appreciate their situation'. In our second interview, Frank described the importance of living close to medical facilities:

> I have had friends that have retired and moved down to the coast onto virgin blocks of land ... going to create this little farmlet that they always dreamed about .... As we get older and in our situation ... we mustn't live too far from the hospital. It's all very well these dream farms and pioneering ... we are better off staying right where we are where we are, not too far from the hospital.

Frank's wife Cindy (60s, spouse with prostate cancer)[7] described this as a source of grief.

> Cindy: I think anyone with cancer suffers a certain amount of grief. Grief for what you used to be and grief for what you know you're not going to be. And you can't do much about that.
>
> R: And is that as the patient and the carer or just ...?
>
> Cindy: Both, because your whole, when you have been married a long time you do everything together.

Rather than realising retirement dreams, cancer limits a couple's capacity to travel or relocate to a removed distance from a hospital. In couples where the cancer had a debilitating impact, doctor's appointments and ill-health got in the way of achieving those plans that couples had made for their future.

---

7   Like Fred and Jane, and Mark and Fiona, I interviewed Frank and Cindy together as they, as a married couple, had taken turns as cancer patient and carer.

For others, cancer did not mean all plans were cancelled. Instead it raised questions about expected future plans. These carers mourned for the taken-for-granted sense of a distant mortality they once had, for their lost sense of a clear life direction that could be anticipated and worked towards, and for the assumptions they had about their futures. To replace these old plans, several carers made new and more immediate plans to accommodate the uncertain future. One couple embarked almost immediately on a three-month holiday around Australia. Another, Linda (40s, spouse with bowel cancer) and her husband, made arrangements to travel interstate in a month to watch a football game.[8]

> We are just going to go down and do something totally stupid. We are going down to see the Wallabies [rugby team] play down in [city] in July. That's how we do it. My brother said, 'I'm going to go. Do you want to come with me?' and I said, 'When is it, July?' 'Yup'. Spur of the moment, we'll go.

Leo and his wife travelled to Europe.

> There are those clichés, live from day to day, make the best of it, and we made it twice to Europe for instance in these last few years. We would again except for the schedule ... of chemotherapy.

Like cancer patients' experiences of liminality (Little et al., 2001), cancer carers' sense of loss is typically characterised by uncertainty and a dual identification with the living and the mourning. Thus grief for the cancer carers in this study did not occur anticipatorily. With so much uncertainty, how could carers achieve anticipatory grief? 'The primary task of mourning is detachment from the lost object' (Whiting and James, 2006: 2). With the future loss being unclear, carers cannot grieve in anticipation of the loss. Instead, many carers experienced indefinite loss, characterised by a heightened awareness of mortality and vagueness about the future which stifled carers' abilities to plan and move forward, prompted them to mourn their possibly lost future plans, reprioritise and make plans only in the immediate future.

Updating Conceptualisations of Loss

In this chapter I examined spouse carers of cancer patients' experiences of loss and grief. While many researchers have examined cancer carer grief in the terminal and bereavement stages, this chapter provides rare qualitative and inductive insight into carers' experiences of loss across the cancer journey. Findings support the existing literature: at the end of their caregiving careers, carers described conventional or anticipatory grief. Building on this literature, this study longitudinally examined

---

8   This is illustrative of what I refer to as being positive but realistic in Chapter 3.

the experiences of carers' at different points within their caregiving careers. Findings indicate that before the end stage of caregiving, carers of a spouse with cancer experienced indefinite loss. Indefinite loss refers to a future loss that is possible but not certain. When their spouses were given life-threatening cancer diagnoses, carers experienced an uncertain loss. Consequently, they grew more aware of their spouse's and their own mortality, they felt static in time and unable to plan for the future; they developed new priorities and mourned their lost taken-for-granted future plans. This type of loss has hitherto been inadequately conceptualised within the literature. Anticipatory grief refers to losses that are certain (Rando, 2000), but indefinite losses are not certain and have not happened. Only one aspect of their indefinite loss had already occurred: a loss of certainty about past laid plans.

In describing this finding, 1) I offer an up-to-date conceptualisation of the loss associated with cancer caregiving to match the conceptualisation of liminality attributed to cancer survivorship; and 2) I build on the anticipatory grief literature, offering a way forward in refining what the concept encompasses.

First, this study is an answer to Fulton and colleague's (1996) call to re-examine loss and grief as medical technology and early detection improve cancer survivorship rates, making cancer patients' futures markedly uncertain. Like cancer patients' experiences of liminality, the sense of loss described by cancer carers in this study was typically characterised by uncertainty. Thus, the term 'indefinite loss' gives a name to cancer carers' particular experiences of loss outside of the terminal or bereavement stage. The finding and name might provide carers with a sense of legitimation. Compiling an overview of cancer carers' loss may lend credibility to their experiences (Bury, 1991). Reading accounts of other carers' emotional struggles can have the comforting effect of preparing carers and decreasing their sense of stigma and isolation (Frank, 1993). Said in another way, people want to know that their experiences are shared by others (Gregory, 2005). Learning about the types of loss carers experience can stop carers from asking 'what is wrong with me?' or 'why am I feeling this way?' The concept indefinite loss makes this contribution, potentially helping carers to feel less alone (Boss, 1999; Sanders et al., 2008; Waldrop, 2007).

The term also has the potential to arm health, support and psychosocial personnel with a clearer means of communicating about and responding to carers of cancer patients' loss. Grief work is now commonly perceived in psychology as a series of tasks, including acknowledging the reality of the loss and closure (Doka, 2006; Kalich and Brabant, 2006). Because the loss is not yet a reality for carers of cancer patients outside of the palliative stage, the approach taken to help carers experiencing indefinite loss might need to be quite different to the approach taken in helping carers experiencing anticipatory or conventional grief.

Second, this concept adds to the literature on anticipatory grief. Studies of anticipatory grief have been widely criticised for their contradictory findings and lack of consistent operational definitions (Al-Gamal and Long, 2010; Fulton et al., 1996; Gilliland and Fleming, 1998; Sweeting and Gilhooly, 1990). Based on the findings presented here, I suggest that much of the confusion surrounding this term is related to the need to clarify the variations in the types of loss that occur. Fulton and colleagues (1996: 1,356) support this assertion: studies need to differentiate 'between grief that is being expressed for past and present [and future] losses .... Previous research has assumed that these time foci are of secondary importance to the emotional response exhibited'. Moreover, it is equally as important to differentiate between losses with different meanings. For example, a loss associated with a spouse's dementia diagnosis may not have the same meaning as a loss associated with a cancer diagnosis. Thus, it would be helpful, in understanding variations of loss and grief, to differentiate between emotional responses to 1) the loss of a social person (e.g. a person with dementia); 2) the loss of a physical person (e.g. a person who has died or gone missing); 3) the imminent loss of a person (e.g. a person in the terminal stages of care); and 4) the uncertain potential loss of a person (e.g. a person diagnosed with a life-threatening illness such as cancer).

The findings presented in this chapter offer conceptual refinement and work towards extending our understanding of loss, as experienced by carers of a spouse with cancer. Further research should help to identify the variation in grief amongst, not only those experiencing certain and uncertain loss, but amongst carers of patients with diverse types of cancer, at various stages and amongst carers with differing relationships to the patient. Past research underscores the importance of using qualitative methodologies in collecting data on grief, to understanding varied processes reflecting constructed realities born from social circumstances (Fulton et al., 1996; Sweeting and Gilhooly, 1990). Studying carers' grief using qualitative methods allows for complexity and avoids the problems of many quantitative studies of imposed operational definitions on carers' experiences (Meuser and Marwit, 2001).

In conclusion, in this chapter I offer a social and participant-driven conceptualisation of cancer carer loss, extending the categories available. In focusing on carers' responses to the loss as well as the meaning of the loss, I offer the term *indefinite loss*. While the concepts conventional grief and anticipatory grief dominate the caregiving literature, these concepts do not resonate with the experiences of contemporary carers of cancer patients providing care outside of the terminal stage. Indefinite loss, grief surrounding a potential future loss, characterised the experiences of most carers in this study. In response to this indefinite loss, carers described a lost taken-for-granted sense of certainty about the future, acute awareness of mortality, reprioritisation of life plans, curtailed ability to plan for the future, and, subsequently, a focus on living in the present. This contribution begins the process of filling a gap in our understanding by describing the lived experiences of cancer carers in a technologically advanced medical age, where cancer and death are no longer synonymous, but the possibility of death is ever-present. Findings also identify many of the causes of confusion in the anticipatory grief literature, highlighting the need to specify the certainty of the loss, when the loss occurs (past, present or future) and the nature of the loss (social or physical) – a finding of particular value to those working with carers of cancer patients.

In the next chapter, I continue to examine carers' emotions. The focus, however, moves away from loss and grief, toward an examination, from psychological and social interactionist perspectives, of carers' coping strategies and emotion work.

Chapter 3

Coping: Managing Hope, Denial or Temporal Anomie?[1]

On a cold and rainy Saturday in May, I used my city map to find Bernard's house. It was located in a quiet suburb around fifteen minutes outside of the city. Bernard (50s) invited me to join him in the living room, where we started the interview by talking about his wife's initial breast cancer diagnosis, mastectomy and terminal recurrence. She died one month before our first interview. Despite his grief, Bernard was eager to be involved in the study, hopeful that sharing his story would be an eventual source of comfort to another carer. Towards the middle of the interview, I asked Bernard about his emotional experience as a carer. He reflected on his most recent caregiving experience, during the recurrence, where his wife was given a relatively clear terminal prognosis. He questioned himself, thoughtfully considering the question, asking if he was in denial. He concluded that he was not:

> I don't believe it was denial of what was happening because that was very clear, so I think it was just to try and keep it out of the major thoughts.

Instead of denial he said it was about consciously focusing on 'the positives' and the present. He said he was a, 'spin doctor that [wa]s trying to put the best spin on the little positives – you would emphasise those and ignore the big negatives'. During our second interview he reflected again on his approach to managing his wife's emotions saying, 'That was something that was not very clear ... what was the right way ... or ... a reasonable way to approach ... what was going on'. He elaborated, explaining that his approach was both 'realistic' and 'positive'.

> Managing this gap between being positive and being realistic .... When you know that you have got three months to live at best, that's realistic .... But again, we didn't sit there with 90 days and mark them off one at a time, right? .... You should be positive. But, [being] positive ... [was not] necessarily in terms of the

---

1   This chapter is a revised and extended version of the following publication (Olson, 2011), reproduced here in accordance with the copyright agreement between the author, Rebecca Olson, and the publisher, Elsevier: Olson, R.E. (2011) Managing Hope, Denial or Temporal Anomie? Informal Cancer Carers' Accounts of Spouses' Cancer Diagnoses. *Social Science & Medicine* 73(6): 904–11. http://www.sciencedirect.com/science/article/pii/S0277953611000426.

outcome of things, they were about a range of peripheral – they were about all the good things that actually happened in the day.

Bernard's reflections illustrate the complexity of carers' emotional responses to their spouses' diagnoses and prognoses. Was his positivity a consequence of being in denial? Or, was it something else?

This chapter examines the emotional impact of a cancer diagnosis on carers of a spouse with cancer. Many psychological studies have examined cancer carers' coping strategies, denial in particular. In this chapter, I examine carers' emotional responses to the diagnosis using psychological and sociological tools, to depict spouses' emotions as located within orientations to time and approaches to prognostication.

Coping strategies are conceptualised in psychology as the 'internal mechanisms' that serve to moderate emotional responses to threatening events such as illness (Frijda, 2000; Remennick, 1998).[2] They are used to decrease the stress of the response through either changing the environment (problem-focused coping) or changing feelings about the situation (emotion-focused coping) (Folkman and Lazarus, 1980; Maex and De Valck, 2006). Emotion-focused coping strategies may include denial, detachment, restraining feelings or avoidance (Carpenter and Miller, 2005; Toseland et al., 1995). Problem-focused coping might include seeking information, assessing the problem, getting guidance and acting or preventing action (Folkman and Lazarus, 1980; Braithwaite, 1990). Studies on caregiving generally find emotion-focused coping strategies to be linked with negative psychological outcomes such as higher rates of anxiety, depression and burden, while problem-focused coping is linked with positive psychological outcomes, such as reduced stress (Carpenter and Miller, 2005; Chambers et al., 2001; Braithwaite, 1990; Saad et al., 1995).

Denial in particular has been found to be problematic to doctor-patient communication and open communication between patients and their families (Bard, 1997; Gear and Haney, 1990; Rose et al., 1997; Sabo, 1990; Stiefel and Razavi, 2006). In the cancer communication and psycho-oncology literature, it is depicted as a widespread and unhealthy coping strategy that should be countered in clinical interactions (Stiefel and Razavi, 2006). Denial refers to the repression or disbelief in a certain reality, such as refusing to believe that someone will die, or disregarding fears that treatment might not work (Dumont and Foss, 1972). Sabo (1990: 80) found that husbands of wives with breast cancer generally avoid discussing their own and their wife's fears. Instead, husbands maintain optimism, which he termed 'paternalistic denial'. Although denial has been shown (in Sabo's and other research) to help carers diminish their own emotional burden, it can frustrate and alienate patients who want to talk about their fears and anxieties (Gear and Haney, 1990; Rose et al., 1997; Sabo, 1990). By denying the seriousness

---

2   See Bury (1991) for a critique of the varied uses of the terms 'coping' and 'strategy' within the chronic illness literature.

of the situation, carers may be indirectly refusing the patient the opportunity to communicate their concerns.

There is, however, doubt about the extent to which denial is employed by carers of cancer patients. Some research emphasises denial as the central coping strategy employed by husbands of wives with breast cancer (Sabo, 1990). Other psychological studies suggest that carers use a number of coping strategies, such as denial, problem-focused coping or normality maintenance, to reduce the impact of a life-altering diagnosis (Nathan, 1990; Rose et al., 1997; Saad et al., 1995). Sociologists have suggested that medical professionals may be perceiving denial where little to none exists, as a *lack* of evidence also 'proves' the existence of denial (Kellehear, 1984: 713). When patients and carers do not talk about grave possibilities implied in their cancer diagnosis they are often perceived by medical professionals to be in denial (Zimmerman, 2007). Thus, the prevalence of denial amongst cancer carers in the psycho-oncology literature is unclear.

In this chapter I offer a sociological analysis of carers' responses to the transformative cancer diagnosis. I use a psychological lens to analyse carers' reported coping strategies first. Following this, I employ an interactionist sociology of emotions lens to provide a complementary sociological understanding of carers' responses to cancer diagnoses. In providing this alternative account, sociologist Arlie Russell Hochschild's (1979) concept of 'emotion work' is central. Her work, developed within the interactionist branch of the sociology of emotions, refers to the manipulation of emotions that people perform on themselves and others to comply with feeling rules or basic cultural norms of how a person should feel in terms of emotional intensity, direction (positive or negative) and duration in a particular situation (Hochschild, 1983; Turner and Stets, 2005). Thomas and colleagues (2001) took this approach in conceptualising the emotions of British cancer patients and carers and found that much of the work that carers do for cancer patients is emotional. Their focus on emotion work also allowed them to perceive patients and carers as more than 'passive victims': as active creators of their cancer experiences (Thomas and Morris, 2002: 181).

Third, after coping and emotion work, I explore the temporal impact of the cancer diagnosis. As illustrated in the previous chapter, diseases like cancer can challenge a cancer patient's and carer's taken-for-granted assumptions about the future. Cancer has the capacity to challenge a patient's and their family's orientation in time (Adam, 1992; Sontag, 1991). Usually, the young, the middle-aged as well as those in the middle- and upper-classes are future-oriented. They are more likely to abstain from indulging in the present to save up their time and money for future enjoyment (Coser and Coser, 1990). The resulting financial security allows them a sense of control and predictability. A cancer diagnosis, however, as Ian's assessment – presented in the last chapter – of saving for retirement as pointless, confronts this sense of control, interrupting the linear perception of a person's biography.

Finally, I analyse carers' descriptions of hearing the diagnosis. The way a medical professional delivers a diagnosis and prognosis can have an immediate emotional affect. It can also shape a patient and carer's shared orientation in time: future- or present-oriented. Collectively, this demonstrates the importance of taking a sociological approach to understanding cancer caregiving – showing the centrality of, not just coping, but emotion work, temporal adjustment and prognostication to carers' experiences.

Coping Strategies

In interviews, I asked carers to tell their story as a cancer carer. Many participants started telling their story by describing the way they responded to hearing the cancer diagnosis and the way it altered their spouse's and their own lives.

Fiona (60s, spouse with prostate cancer) and Andrew (60s, spouse with breast cancer), for example, described fears about their partner's death as their immediate reaction. Fiona said, 'When you first hear … the word [cancer], I think most people have a negative reaction …. You normally leap to "well, hopefully it's not terminal"'. The prognosis for Andrew's wife was more certainly bleak. He said the diagnosis 'crystallises the finality of things … you know that [life is restricted] … – it's a hit … that there is a finite time for [my wife]'. The diagnosis prompted them to realise life's brevity.

I also asked participants how they reacted to the diagnosis and how they approached or dealt with the emotional side of caregiving. Analysis of their responses suggests that spouse cancer carers may not use denial as a coping strategy as often as some of the literature suggests. Carers experienced a range of emotions that denial would circumvent: anger, anxiety, depression, fear, guilt, frustration and sadness. The accounts of Mitch, Anne, Blake, as well as Bernard's story – presented at the beginning of this chapter – illustrate carers' awareness of their spouses' indefinite futures.

Mitch (50s), whose wife was diagnosed with breast cancer a few months before our first interview, told me about his rarely articulated, but clear awareness that his wife's future was uncertain.

> One thing [my wife] has made clear: no plans …. This year we were watching the State of Origin [rugby] game and I said, 'How about next year we go?' and she looked up and said, 'I could be dead by then'. We don't talk a lot. I just give [my wife] time and I am here.

In our second interview, following surgery and radiotherapy, Anne (30s, spouse with glandular cancer), introduced in Chapter 2, said that she and her husband work to not think about a recurrence or the possibility that he may die.

> We try very hard to … say we can't think about it … because then you don't focus on everything else day to day. You don't focus on the good things. You focus on the negatives.

She and her husband were both clearly aware of the gravity and uncertainty of her husband's diagnosis, but to reintegrate with the living, working and parenting world, it was necessary to control their anxiety by bracketing off their thoughts of his cancer.

Blake's (40s) wife was diagnosed with aggressive metastatic breast cancer before our first interview and died a month before our second interview. He said during our first meeting:

> You don't want to think about it, we hope that she doesn't die ... I really need her a lot. And she doesn't want to die now. No one wants to die, but we don't [know]. We are just hoping for the best. So I am trying to keep her spirits up and just hope.

Like Anne, it was clear to Blake that the future was uncertain, but focusing on the possibilities and the present made it easier to function day to day.

It is clear that these carers, whether their partner's prognosis was certain or uncertain, were well aware and acknowledged the gravity of their circumstances and, thus, were not in denial. The positive approach adopted by many carers, which could be misinterpreted as denial, was actually a direct response to a carer's awareness of the disease's gravity and the uncertainty of their spouse's future.

Instead of denial, carers seemed to use a range of coping strategies. Distraction was the approach most widely employed. More than half of the carers in this study (18 of 32) reported using this technique to push their mind onto other thoughts and away from their fears and anxieties surrounding their spouse's diagnosis. To keep from always focusing on the cancer, these carers plunged into 'busy work' (Judy, 60s, spouse with asbestos-related cancer), paid work, housework, holiday planning or exercise. When I asked Kyle (40s, spouse with breast cancer), for instance, about how he approached the emotional side of caring he replied, 'I buried myself in work and things to do .... Just [to] keep my mind busy, lots of puzzles'.

A quarter (8 of 32) of the carers interviewed compartmentalised or 'shelved' (Fiona, 60s, spouse with prostate cancer) their thoughts and worries while caring, for fear that focusing on the resulting feelings would inhibit their ability to provide care. Sally's (40s) husband was diagnosed with muscle invasive bladder cancer. During our first interview, she explained:

> I don't think I deal with it [emotions] at all. I think maybe it is just being put aside somewhere in a little bubble to be (laughs) dealt with at a later time .... I am actually aware of the fact that I don't deal with it, it's too hard (laughs).

During our second interview she elaborated further:

> I don't do a lot of talking about emotions … I don't consciously think about it …
> I don't spend a lot of [time on emotions] … . It's partly that … if you delve into
> the emotional and it doesn't resolve in a way, then you are in a mess.[3]

Four of the thirty-two interviewees reported using escapist coping strategies such as drinking or gambling to help them momentarily forget the diagnosis and corresponding uncertainty. Leo (60s, spouse with breast cancer) said, 'I drink more. I started smoking a few times again … self-indulgences'. Carlie (50s, spouse with oral cancer) used gambling as an escape. 'I have an out once a week and go and play the pokie machines (laughs). And I always call that my … therapy'. Charlie (50s, spouse with breast cancer) used both: 'I drank a lot for a while … . Going down to the pub … played the pokies'. Other strategies, reported by only a few carers, included taking anti-anxiety medication, meditating, expressing emotions to friends and family, avoiding information on the disease, distancing oneself from the patient, taking action to address problems and finding 'happy outcomes to things that are distressing' (Kyle, 40s, spouse with breast cancer), what Hochschild (1983) refers to as cognitive emotion management. These strategies were not mutually exclusive. Most carers reported temporarily using more than one coping strategy throughout their caring careers, in different situations. What was consistent, however, was the effort to manage their own and their spouses' emotions to be positive.

Emotion Work

Coping strategies varied, but all participants, to differing extents, reported doing emotion work. Their emotions were not just experienced as being solely about themselves. Carers actively tried to change not only their own emotions but also their spouse's emotions to conform to culturally defined 'feeling rules' and 'good patient' display rules (Small, 1996: 267).[4] Carers' definitions of the good patient centred around being positive and stoic. Carers were proud of spouses who were emotionally 'strong' instead of down (Sally, 40s, spouse with bladder cancer; Tyler, 60s, spouse with haematological cancer). Carers regarded highly those spouses who showed bravery during medical procedures, in facing the public and in facing death. Anne (30s, spouse with glandular cancer), for example, spoke with awe about her husband's bravery at returning to work, despite his ongoing radiotherapy and being disfigured. Tyler said his wife's 'strength of mind', approach to patienthood as a patient with an incurable haematological cancer and

---

3   See Chapter 5 for further insight into the temporal dimensions of Sally's carer story.

4   Davis and George's (1993: 171) review of the literature shows that definitions of a 'good patient' by hospital workers vary, but overall, good patients are those who cooperate with and are pleasant to staff, maintain motivation, avoid complaining and do not consume too much of medical staff's time.

her matter of fact decision to stop dialysis and die was impressive and a relief. He said she never showed any 'histrionics', she was 'realistic', 'courageous and dignified'. He reflected on his caregiving experience concluding, 'Had she been a person who cried out in the middle of the night, "Why me?", I would have no doubt … a totally [different] approach'. Leo (60s, spouse with breast cancer), who was both a medical doctor and carer, spoke about this in the most depth.

> When she was really really sick in the hospital everybody was saying what a nice lady she is because … she was so polite and pleasant and cooperative. Model patient. So, I was proud of her, we all were … . If you [the patient] are really hideous … it would be harder. That would separate the saints from the mortals.

A 'bad patient', as Leo indicated, was one who did not cooperate, show bravery or positivity; one who 'throws in the towel and gives up hope' (Joe, 60s, spouse with ovarian cancer; Judy, 60s, spouse with asbestos-related cancer; Cindy, 60s, spouse with prostate cancer; Frank, 70s, spouse with haematological cancer); 'gives up the ghost and lies in bed or moans about things' (Joe); or 'throws their bum in the corner' (Judy) (a boxing euphemism). Frank and Cindy, for instance, an older couple who had taken turns as carer and patient, repeatedly said that patients should not dwell on the negatives; they should not 'drop their bundle' and become reclusive 'voluntary vegetables' who wallow in their depression and watch television all day. Bad patients were the ones who focused on their fears and remorse, did not manage their own emotions and cried loudly in despair.

One reason for defining bad patients this way was because of the amount of emotion work involved for the carer. Brave and positive patients were said to be easier to care for. As Tyler (60s, spouse with haematological cancer) explained, '90 per cent' of caring is emotion work.

> We have seen … what happens to people who can't cope and … that is terrible for the carer … . It is terrible for the patient obviously, but when somebody … is looking after somebody who is depressed … says, 'it's not worth it' … that must be an awful situation.

In other words, when a patient manages his or her own emotions to comply with social and hospital feeling rules, a carer's job is a lot easier. When patients accepted cancer and uncertainty bravely, this was considered a particular relief for carers and family.

However, not all patients were able to stay this positive and brave. Mark (60s, spouse with breast cancer), who had experience as both a patient and carer, illustrates this point. As a prostate cancer patient, he vacillated between periods of depression and outbursts where he flew 'off the handle' at his wife, Fiona, because he was frustrated about his incontinence following surgery. 'Scan anxiety' was another commonly cited reason for patients' angry outbursts. Several carers, whose partners were required to get scans every few months to monitor the status of their tumours, said their partners had severe anxiety before their scan results which prompted their anger. Linda (40s, spouse with bowel cancer), for instance, said her husband:

> Gets really cranky and hard to live with during that period when we are waiting for a result …. You think … 'You are being absolutely ridiculous. I would quite happily strangle you. That would solve everything'. Of course you don't mean it, and he is sweetness and light the minute he gets the result, if it's a good result.

Therefore, carers saw the bulk of their role as helping their spouse to work at being a model and stoical patient: 'It is the emotional part that becomes the greater challenge' (Rodney, 30s, spouse with breast cancer). To manage their spouse's emotions, carers employed a number of techniques. These included: distraction, pep talks, listening, acting, lying and blocking undesired communication. Carers distracted patients by getting them to 'focus on something else' such as travel plans or facilitating speedy treatment to curtail any prolonged uncertain introspection (Fiona, 60s, spouse with prostate cancer). They emotionally buoyed patients during depression, difficult treatment and even difficulty in eating by giving pep talks, saying 'we can beat this' (Jane, 60s, spouse with prostate cancer; Marian, 50s, spouse with neurological cancer) and 'you can do this' (Anne, 30s, spouse with glandular cancer). They helped their spouses to 'deal with [their] fears' by encouraging the patient to talk to them and/or a counsellor or support group (Rodney).

Many carers reported concealing feelings of distress from their spouse or leading the patient to believe that the family was financially and emotionally stable when this was not the case to keep the patient from worrying about anything other than him or herself. Linda (40s, spouse with bowel cancer) put on an 'award-winning act' of hopefulness for her husband. A couple of carers even blocked communication from friends and family who were perceived to be too negative or not sufficiently focused on the patient. Matthew (30s, spouse with breast cancer), for example, said, 'Some ring up with their personal problems and unload onto [my wife] …. I filter these people'.

It became clear that in the views of the spouses I interviewed, a carer's role was to help their partner to be positive and brave again when patients deviated from the emotional displays expected of a model patient. Carers varied, however, in their approaches to being positive at a time when there were so many reasons to be negative. Bernard (50s, spouse with breast cancer) became a 'spin-doctor' focusing on positives from the day, but acknowledging his wife's limited future. Other carers felt optimistic and wanted their friends to be optimistic too. Blake (40s, spouse with breast cancer), for instance, asked of a friend who did not know what to say during a phone call, 'can't he say she's going to be alright?' He wanted his friends to help him to be positive. Linda (40s, spouse with bowel cancer), however, got annoyed when friends were overly optimistic about her husband's future. She wanted friends to 'acknowledge' that 'things aren't going to be alright'; that her husband was not likely to survive. To understand why carers' approaches to emotion management were so varied, I re-examined the transcripts with the following question in mind: how do carers and patients maintain hope? I found that carers' and patients' orientations towards time were key elements in how they managed.

Temporal Anomie

Many spouse carers of cancer patients reported a lack of control and lost direction in time as a consequence of the diagnosis.[5] Matthew (30s, spouse with breast cancer), for instance, said 'it is not winning or losing the battle against cancer, it's learning to live with it'. Their spouses' diagnosis curtailed their ability to plan for holidays, future careers and financial decisions. Mitch, (50s, spouse with breast cancer), quoted earlier, was unable to make plans to see a rugby game the following year. Linda, quoted in Chapter 2, was unable to make career and financial plans because it involved thinking too far into an uncertain future. Linda (40s, spouse with bowel cancer) asked herself, 'Should I buy a house that would be more suited to a single person?' and then berated herself mentally for planning a life without her spouse.

This hindered ability to plan left many carers feeling confused and guilty, in a temporal position of stasis. In addition to being a feature of indefinite loss, I conceptualise this here as *temporal anomie*: a challenged orientation towards time based on the prolific sociologist Emile Durkheim's use of the term 'anomie' to describe the sense of normlessness and lost direction that people experience after major events such as an economic depression (Collins and Makowsky, 1998: 110).[6]

To overcome this temporal anomie many carers adopted an alternative approach to time. To address their sense of interruption and purposelessness towards the future, patients and carers either 1) readjusted their temporal orientation to be present-oriented or 2) performed cognitive emotion-work to reinterpret their perception of the cancer diagnosis and maintain a future-oriented perspective.

Positive but Realistic

Couples who became present-oriented called this being 'positive but realistic'. These or similar words were repeated in 17 interviews by carers or couples where the cancer patient was facing a terminal prognosis. These carers, as illustrated by

---

5   See Chapter 2 on indefinite loss.

6   Mellor (1992: 13), in an article that builds a case for a sociology of death, similarly argues that, 'The existential confrontation with death, one's own or the death of others, has the potential to ... call into question the meaningfulness and reality of the social frameworks in which they participate, shattering their [a person's] ontological security'.

Bernard who was introduced at the start of this chapter, focused on the uplifting or pleasant occurrences each day instead of focusing on the loss that lay ahead. They were well aware and accepting of their spouses' (potentially) limited futures, but felt compelled to be positive about something: the time they had with their spouse in the present.[7] Blake (40s, spouse with breast cancer), for instance, said 'you are not at the funeral ... there is still living to do'. Judy (60s, spouse with asbestos-related cancer) described this as focusing on 'now'.

> I don't say to him, 'Look, this is going to kill you'. I don't say that. I am pretty sure he knows it. So I don't think we talk into the future; I am sure we don't. We just talk about now. We deal with now and it makes you look at now more than you ever did before.

Linda (40s, spouse with bowel cancer) described being positive but realistic as the best approach because if she were to go too far in either direction (being sure of a cure and optimistic or being sure of the loss and depressed) she thought it would be too difficult to change her direction. She did, however, have occasional doubts, saying 'it's a bit like correcting course in a sailing ship ... . Do I need to correct my course a little bit?' She sought confirmation from a nurse educator that this was 'the correct' approach for her to take.

> I said to her ... 'I am not sure if my perspective is the right perspective' ... . She said, 'No, you have actually got the right perspective, unlike many of the other people we deal with. You have got two extreme reactions a lot of the time. One is there is no hope no matter what we do ... . Then you have got the other ones who think because they have had this treatment that it's a guaranteed miracle cure' ... . She said, 'You have got the right perspective. You know we are not giving you any guarantees ... you are just forging ahead and ... enjoy[ing] what you have now. That's where we would like our patients [and carers] to be'.

While only one participant in this study adopted the 'no hope' perspective presented by the nurse educator, just over half adopted the 'right perspective': being positive but realistic. Several others took on what the nurse described as overly optimistic.

Optimistic

Instead of adapting to a present-focused orientation, six carers remained focused on the future by believing they would beat the cancer, typically as part

---

7   Recently bereaved carers in Duke's (1998: 833) study similarly described trying to 'make the best of the time they had together' with the patient.

of a complementary or alternative medicine (CAM)[8] regime that emphasises the 'interdependence of the organism's biological, mental, and emotional manifestations' (Capra, 1982: 380). Marian (50s, spouse with neurological cancer), for example, followed CAM recommendations: spending hours in the kitchen making organic foods and buying over $1,000 worth of Chinese herbal medicine. As noted in Chapter 2, taking this approach, however, was not easy for her.

> If you go down that path you have to truly believe that you can beat it, which for me was a general dichotomy because … all my sort of logic is to go with the odds … my background was in Science …. But the other part of you … goes down the [optimistic path], gets the Chinese medicine, we went to Ian Gawler's meditation for healing workshop.

To maintain their future-orientation, Marian had to do cognitive emotion work to stay optimistic and convince herself and her husband that he would survive.

Carers who incorporated these CAM recommendations into their future-oriented and optimistic approach explained that it allowed them to feel more in control and gave them 'something to do' (Anne, 30s, spouse with glandular cancer). For Rodney (30s, spouse with breast cancer), being optimistic was the basis of the support that he provided to his wife. He described it as one of the few 'weapons' he had in his wife's fight with cancer and went on to say:

> I guess that has … been my [approach], without going over the top and with pom poms and music … it has just [been] … gentle encouragement and at other times, more forward …. An active positive persistent encouragement.

Rodney described this as both a preference and an act that required vigilance, describing his optimism as wanting to:

> Bury my head in the sand and think everything is okay …. Focus on the upside and not let the downside influence or shape me …. I would much rather be focusing on the positives and be optimistic … rather than dwell in fear of losing her early and not having the opportunity to grow old with her.

For Rodney, however, agreeing to be optimistic with his wife was a source of guilt. While he was consciously trying to believe his wife would survive, thoughts about her possible death crept into his subconscious, causing him to feel unfaithful.

> I would wake up in the middle of the night preparing [my wife's] eulogy and then feeling guilty for … almost giving up on her. Or I found in making investment

---

8   Complementary means in addition to, while alternative means instead of Western medicine (Tovey et al., 2007).

decisions, well hang on we can't really rely on [my wife's] income and then feeling guilty for even thinking that.[9]

This was an ongoing source of guilt for Rodney. By our second interview he described it as 'the great dilemma' which 'remains in my mind, in my heart ... when I find myself subconsciously ... giving the eulogy or thinking about my daughter and I if [my wife] dies'. Their optimistic approach also negated his desire to talk about death with his wife, making it impracticable for him to ask questions that would challenge his wife's positive determination.

> I don't know how many times I have thought about this. Each time I have decided not to raise it .... I don't know if – when she eventually dies ... whether she wants to be buried or cremated .... I am ... reluctant to raise that with her now .... I am worried about the effects that that would have on [my wife].

Normalcy

Eight carers did not change their time-orientation, nor did they start believing they would beat the cancer. Instead, these carers did cognitive emotion work to counter their fears that anything was different. Two carers who adopted this approach were facing a prognosis that was not terminal, where high success rates had been predicted. For two much older couples, the likelihood of death was becoming a reality, and little cognitive emotion work was required. For the other four, the threat posed by the cancer was years in the past. Along the way they had done emotion work to re-join the future-oriented, 'normal' world. Patrick (50s, spouse with breast cancer), for example, did this by continuously describing death as a certainty of life.

> I work on the principal that sooner or later we are all going to die and most of us don't know when it is going to be .... Don't go hanging around the place being like a stale bottle .... I might get hit by a bus tomorrow too and that could be fatal .... We had taken the deliberate path that we were going to make things work normally, as normal as possible .... Get on with the treatment and see what happens. If it don't work, well [she] was out for the count anyway, so that would be it .... Death is inevitable .... At the end of the day, what people would like to know is cancer is slow; a bullet is very quick.

Using the premise that death is inevitable, he argued that his wife's cancer diagnosis did not change anything. He and his wife encouraged each other and their children to carry on as usual and continue 'looking forward' and 'plan[ning]

---

9   See also Chapter 2 on indefinite loss.

for the future'.[10] Mitch (50s, spouse with breast cancer) and his wife also adopted this approach to the future, but to a lesser extent. He said that Melanie felt 'a little bit disappointed that she [couldn't] ... do some things' and occasionally expressed fear that she might not have a future. In general, however, Mitch and Melanie felt they needed to 'get on with life. I have got kids to worry about, I have got plans'. They saw cancer and treatment as a 'process' that they had to go through as part of life.

Medical Professionals' Influence

Carers and patients seemed to select these frameworks (positive but realistic, optimistic or 'normal') in conjunction with or in opposition to the way their spouse's diagnosis and prognosis were delivered. Diagnosis and prognosis are often conflated in cancer studies because statistics are inexact (Gould, 1995; Little, 1995). This leaves room for medical professionals to frame carers' and patients' perceptions of their uncertain future. Carers talked about the delivery of their spouse's cancer diagnosis and other conversations with doctors and nurses as important in shaping or evaluating their outlook. Linda (50s, spouse with breast cancer), quoted earlier, for instance, asked a nurse educator if her 'positive but realistic' approach was the right approach. The delivery (or ongoing deliveries in the cases of remission, recurrence or metastasis) of the diagnosis and prognosis, in particular, seemed to be influential in shaping a couple's approach to the future. Informing patients and carers of the statistical prognosis provided an opportunity for medical staff to present the technical and statistical jargon in a specific light for the couple.

The imprecise nature of statistical data and difficulty in translating 'frequential probabilities' of a population into a prediction about one patient's likely response to treatment and disease is what makes addressing temporal orientation so central to interactions within oncology (Little, 1995). As Little (1995: 20–21) explains, 'the clinician may know precisely the probability of a diagnosis and the likelihood of a cure with a certain treatment, but cannot know the outcome of the individual'. In addition to statistical data being difficult to apply to a specific patient's situation, it can also be difficult for the patient and carer to understand these statistics (Gould, 1995). Therefore, telling patients and carers the statistical information on its own is insufficient. Little (1995) likens it to drawing marbles from a bag: 'at best, [clinicians] can express their conviction ... as being equivalent to a conviction that they will draw a red marble from a bag containing 70 black marbles and 30 red ones. Guillemin (1997: 76) also criticises this tactic, describing it as 'little better than offering a lottery ticket to someone who is destitute'. Thus, doctors must guide patients in how they should feel about their prognosis (Small, 1996). They must frame statistical prognoses

---

10   Bury (1991) reports similar findings.

within temporal re-orientations to clarify their meaning and, at the same time, ensure patients do not become too depressed.

For patients and carers, hearing the cancer diagnosis was said to be visceral and memorable. Carers vividly recounted how they reacted to the diagnosis. Andrew (cited earlier) described the diagnosis of a recurrence as a 'hit'. Mitch (50s, spouse with breast cancer) said the diagnosis 'shook' his wife. Many others described it as a 'shock' (Bernard, 50s, spouse with breast cancer; Carlie, 50s, spouse with oral cancer; Charlie, 50s, spouse with breast cancer; Cindy, 60s, spouse with prostate cancer; Leo, 60s, spouse with breast cancer; Millicent, 60s, spouse with haematological cancer). Thus, the delivery of the diagnosis was the opportune time for medical professionals, knowingly or otherwise, to frame and guide patients' and carers' temporal orientations and subsequent emotions. A medical professional's casting of a diagnosis and prognosis was said to range from certainly bleak to slow and ongoing to probable survival.

Certainly Bleak

Anne and her husband, for instance, were given a bleak prognosis in a startling manner. They went to see their GP after months of putting it off and they were referred to a surgeon, who may have consequently felt obligated to berate Anne and her husband into taking his cancer more seriously. Despite the contradictions in the literature on the prevalence of denial amongst cancer patients and carers (Docherty, 2004; McNamara, 2001), Zimmermann (2007) asserts that medical professionals regularly perceive denial and actively work to counter it. Literature on communication in oncology shows that denial is believed to be prevalent and a danger to open communication. If the patient appears to be in denial, clinicians are instructed to 'underline ... that the medical situation is serious' (Stiefel and Razavi, 2006: 43). The surgeon, possibly following this advice, did so by repeatedly telling Anne and her husband that they were too late, there was nothing more to do. As Anne (30s, spouse with glandular cancer) explained:

> We went into the office and [the surgeon] looked at all the test results and just sort of said to us, 'well you are too late. That is it; there is nothing you can do. You are going to die rah rah rah' .... He said, 'it is very very bad' and asked us if we had life insurance for him and, he just wrote him off.

Thus, in Anne's experience, the surgeon not only delivered the statistical prognosis information, but did so in a way that challenged their future-orientation. Although Anne said that this way of framing the diagnosis had the effect of blaming them for the cancer's advanced stage,[11] their subsequent re-orientation to be present-

---

11   According to Davis and George (1993: 260) this is very common. In their words, 'each consultation can potentially go either of two ways: blame and short shrift for bringing something trivial, or blame for delaying consultation'.

focused helped them to be positive about smaller achievements such as surviving surgery (after they found a surgeon who would operate), eating and drinking normally and withstanding radiation.

Graduated Prognosis

For Sally (40s, spouse with bladder cancer) and her husband, the prognosis and re-orientation process was less abrupt, much slower and less certain. She said:

> There is a trickle feed of information .... They tell you so much at one stage, and then when the results aren't good, the wording subtly but significantly changes and it's a consistent change .... [Phrases like] 'muscle invasive' ... it's just this new phrase that you weren't entitled to before.

This is what is referred to in the oncology communication literature as 'partial' (Surbone, 2006: 95) or 'graduated' disclosure (Field and Copp 1999; as cited in Kennedy and Lloyd-Williams, 2006: 48). Mamo (1999: 26) asserts that this is often necessary as many patients and family members need time to absorb the emotionally laden prognosis. The doctor, according to the legal and oncological communication literature, needs to judge how much information the patient can handle in each consultation (Skene, 1990). If patients are 'loaded' down with too much information on possible outcomes, they might become overwhelmed and lose hope (Stiefel and Razavi, 2006: 40).

For Sally's husband, medical staff started with a more optimistic approach, neglecting to mention the statistical likelihood of a recurrence and abstaining from talk about the patient's increased risk of recurrence elsewhere after radiation. Sally concluded that this approach did keep her husband positive before surgery and radiation, possibly increasing his chances of success, but, it left her to 'pick up the pieces' afterwards. She had to continually (re)manage her husband's outlook and associated emotions. Unlike Anne's experience, where their positive outlook on the future was immediately rejected, but slowly reintroduced, Sally's experience was one of ongoing temporal anomie. Because medical staff were positive to the point of withholding information until negative results forced them to slowly present a less positive outlook, Sally subsequently lost trust in medical staff and was unsure of what approach to the future she should take.[12] The surgeon told her after removing the cancerous organ that cancer 'should be a thing of the past'. But, as a result of the changes in their roles and priorities and as a result of the multiple temporal orientations they had adopted, Sally was sceptical, saying, 'I don't know if it can ever be that sort of thing'.

---

12 Little (1995: 19) asserts that language hinders clear communication in the clinical setting. With patients using lay language and doctors using jargon, there are 'innumerable misapprehensions working on both sides of the consultation'. Thus, the medical staff's reluctance may not be the only impetus behind graduated prognoses.

Positive

Other carers talked about doctors encouraging patients and carers to adopt a more positive outlook. For those patients whose prognosis was terminal, doctors tried to help carers and patients to be more positive, not about their future, but about their time in the present. They said things like 'she is not dead yet' (Blake, 40s, spouse with breast cancer) or organised for scans to be postponed to allow the patient and the carer to travel and enjoy 'the now' (Linda, 40s, spouse with bowel cancer). One oncologist said, "'Try to forget that you have got it. Try to carry on with your life"' (Judy, 60s, spouse with asbestos-related cancer). For those patients whose prognosis was survival for the foreseeable future, doctors were said to have helped the carer and patient to take a 'normal' approach and be more positive about the future. To this end, they relayed statistics on the combined treatment's higher success rates and encouraged carers and patients to live as usual – that is to live and plan with the future in mind. Mitch's (50s, spouse with breast cancer) wife's oncologist, for example, provided them with a statistical schema for thinking of their future as all but certain.

> The oncologist … draws a little line … and says, 'Okay, we start off here, and we are working towards … as close as we can get to a 100 per cent cure …. Mastectomy … that has given you a 50 to 60 per cent cure …. Intensive chemotherapy … that will give another 20 per cent, so that is 70 to 80 per cent …. I will do another three months of less invasive … chemotherapy followed by about eight months of Herceptin … that will give you upwards of another 20 per cent. So on those figures you can get between 90 and 100 per cent'.

These findings show that carers do emotion work that is directly linked to diagnostication and prognostication. Carers do not just cope or perform ongoing emotion work of their own volition; they do so in response to cultural feeling rules related to being a 'good patient', CAM guidelines and the way medical staff frame diagnostic and prognostic information.

Cancer Carer Emotions: A Sociological Approach

The insights presented here apply interactionist theories on emotion to understanding cancer carers' emotional experiences, providing a complementary lens to the largely psychological literature on cancer caregiving to date. First, these findings highlight the limitations of adopting a singularly psychological approach to understanding carers' experiences, suggesting the need for a more encompassing lens. Denial provides a rich example. In the cancer communication and psycho-oncology literature, denial is reportedly widespread (Stiefel and Razavi, 2006; Zimmerman, 2007; Sabo, 1990). As the quotes presented here indicate, denial does not fully encapsulate carers of cancer patients' emotional experiences. It is possible that some carers are in denial, and these carers chose not to participate in this study. The accounts presented here, however, suggest that interaction norms of not focusing on death may have been mistaken as denial in past research. The experiences of Mitch, Anne, Blake and Bernard indicate that carers who avoid talking about cancer may be adhering to interaction norms where discussions on death are categorised as taboo (Elias, 1985; Jalland, 2006; Wilkinson and Kitzinger, 2000), or at the very least unpleasant. Preferring to avoid the awkwardness, emotional eruption and interruption that might follow (Kellehear, 1984), carers may actively silence these conversations. Furthermore, carers in this study employed a range of coping strategies.

The popularity of individualistic examinations of carers' coping strategies may result in the misdiagnosis and over diagnosis of denial. Before looking for an individual and psychologistic origin in studies on carers' emotional experiences and challenges, future inquiries should first rule out the multi-factorial influences that are likely shaping carers' emotion work. This will improve the quality of cancer caregiving researchers' recommendations about how best to support carers, as the level of inquiry shapes a study's recommendations. If, for example, carers are found to be employing unhelpful (to themselves or the patient) coping strategies, then the problem is seen to be located in 'the psychological make-up' of the carer (Thomas and Morris, 2002: 181). Readily available therapy might then be appropriate. If, on the other hand, carers are found to be performing unhelpful emotion work (on themselves and the patients in their care), the problem is seen to be 'rooted in the social management of cancer', in the cultural and medical system norms that guide a carer's emotion work (Thomas and Morris, 2002: 181). The scope for change resulting from this kind of finding might include the carer as well as medical professionals, counsellors and wider cultural norms.

Adopting a sociological lens further highlights the importance of context to understanding carers' emotional experiences. While there is debate within the psychology of emotions as to the ideal level of analysis, biological, cognitive or socio-cultural (Frijda, 2000: 61), in sociology the reflective nature of our interactions is widely acknowledged. People's perceptions of themselves and their subsequent emotional reactions are shaped by their assessments of what others think (Mead, 2000; Hochschild, 1979; Small, 1996; Stocker and Hegeman, 1996). An interactionist sociology of emotions approach to understanding carers' emotions as emotion work, and to understanding this emotion work as organised by a temporal re-orientation, provides rich insight into carers' and patients' reactions to cancer diagnoses. Diagnosis and prognosis do not solely lead to denial or other forms of coping, but to an active engagement with emotions over time. Interactions with medical professionals form the basis from which carers and patients understand the impact of the diagnosis (or diagnoses) and then shape their own and their spouse's emotions. Thus, interactionist sociological conceptualisations of emotions could complement, if not replace, the individualistic psycho-oncology focus on coping strategies (Thomas et al., 2001).

Second, the insights into cancer carers' emotions presented here, using a sociological imagination, show that in addition to coping, carers also manage their own and their spouse's emotions to comply with 'good patient' feeling rules of being stoical and positive. Based on analysis of this finding, I offer a clearer distinction between the psychological concept 'coping strategy' and the sociological concept 'emotion work'. Coping strategies, such as distraction and escapism, are employed in the short-term. Many are used, not just one consistently, to temporarily avoid the emotions, such as fear and anxiety, surrounding the cancer diagnosis. Emotion work, in contrast, is performed on oneself and others (Emslie et al., 2009). Unlike coping, carers together with their spouses, do *ongoing* emotion work to conform to ('good patient' and 'good carer') expectations, feeling rules and a specific temporal-orientation.

Third, employing theories from sociological studies of time to this analysis reveals the centrality of time to understanding cancer carers' emotion work. Planning is a 'key modern organisational and psychological feature', particularly for the young and middle-class (Lewis and Weigart, 1990: 94). It allows for a sense of control and predictability. The temporal disruption of a cancer diagnosis can prompt a person to lose their ability to plan and lose their sense of control, what I refer to as *temporal anomie*. Adding to the few sociology of emotions studies that link time and emotion (Fung and Carstensen, 2006; Hochschild, 2000), these findings show that this biographical disruption intersects with a couples' attempts to manage emotions, producing a complex situation where carer and patient perform emotion work to redefine their focus or temporal orientation. To address their consequent sense of interruption and purposelessness towards time, carers either adjust their temporal scope to be present-oriented or perform cognitive emotion-work to reinterpret their perception of the cancer diagnosis and maintain a future-oriented perspective. This redefinition is prompted by the cancer diagnosis and the context in which it is delivered by medical professionals. Thus, patients and carers experience temporal anomie as a consequence of hearing a diagnosis and prognosis.

Fourth, this chapter shows the importance of the casting of the diagnosis to carers' temporal orientation and emotion work. Giving a grim, gradual or probable survival prognosis shaped carers' temporally guided emotion work. Maintaining 'hope' currently dominates the oncology diagnosis communication literature (Surbone, 2006; Salander and Moynihan, 2010), but the insights presented here offer a more specific conceptualisation of what medical professionals do when they deliver a diagnosis. Hope is quite ambiguous. Reviews of the literature show multiple and conflicting definitions (Kennedy and Lloyd-Williams, 2006; Miller, 2007). Some link hope to goals (Dufault and Martocchio, 1985), others to life purpose (Owen, 1989), 'time refocusing', 'spiritual beliefs', 'uplifting energy' (Herth, 1993: 542) and a sense of 'inner strength' (Benzein and Saveman, 1998: 10). Instead of using the term 'hope', I suggest that addressing a patients' and carers' temporal anomie more directly communicates what physicians, and other medical professionals such as nurses, in this study were said to do in clinical narratives: re-cast or encourage patients and carers to assume certain orientations to time (Frankenberg, 1992; White, 2006).

Overall, this chapter builds on the groundwork laid by Thomas and colleagues (2001) for thinking about cancer carers' emotions from social and sociological perspectives, rather than solely individualistic and psychological perspectives. It demonstrates the interactionist nature of carers' emotions. Their emotions are not purely responses to a diagnosis outside of their control (Thomas and Morris, 2002). Denial does not fully represent carers of cancer patients' emotional responses to a cancer diagnosis. Carers also do emotion work. While carers cope with overwhelming fears and anxieties in the short-term using strategies such as distraction, in the long-term they manage their own and their spouses' emotions to comply with cultural expectations around being a good patient and re-orient their positivity in time (positive about the future or the time left in the present) in response to the temporal anomie that the diagnosis prompts. The diagnostic process (Jutel and Dew, 2014) and the light in which the prognosis is cast by medical professionals (imminent death, gradual or survival) plays an important role in informing carers' emotion management, highlighting the social nature of the emotion work that carers do. Carers' temporally specific emotion work is guided by cultural feeling rules, medical professionals' advice, literature (such as the CAM literature) that may counter this advice and medical professional's casting of the diagnosis.

This suggests the fruitfulness of widening the scope of inquiry. There is little understanding in this literature of cancer carers' and patients' experiences as the result of many interactions, internal, financial, social, medical and otherwise. A sociological approach to understanding cancer caregiving includes the influence of medical professionals' categorisations of emotional responses, the impact of prominent (CAM and other) literature and of social support on carers and patients' emotional and mental health, instead of continuing to examine carers', patients' or couples' coping strategies alone. As it has been demonstrated here, emotions are interactive. Carers' and patients' emotions do not just exist in a 'dyad' (Rose et al., 1997: 131) or even a 'triad' (Kearney et al., 2007: 21) that includes the patient, carer and doctor. Nurse educators (as Linda's experience shows), nurses (Hunt, 1991), psychologists, other members of a multidisciplinary care team and the power relations between these members (Allen et al., 2004), as well as family, friends, and culture (Emslie et al., 2009; Surbone, 2006) all influence patients' and carers' emotional experiences of diagnosis and cancer.

In the next chapter, the importance of adopting a sociological framework in understanding cancer caregiving is built further. Carer's emotional confusion is examined from an interactionist theoretical basis, revealing the conflict between spouse and carer feeling rules.

Chapter 4

Feeling: Prognosis Ambiguity, Role Conflict and Emotion Work in Cancer Caregiving[1]

Matthew's (40s) wife was diagnosed with aggressive breast cancer six weeks before our interview. When we met, he was feeling anger towards the cancer. '[I] get very angry because I tend to think .... "How can this happen? Why?"' He was frustrated from 'wearing 15 different hats'. Following his wife's diagnosis and subsequent treatment, their roles had changed: 'I come home from work, I do dinner, I do the housework, she does what she can ... I have taken over all the finances'. He wanted to talk to his wife about his feelings of fear, frustration and anger, but his role as caregiver prevented him from doing so, illustrating the contradictions in the expectations associated with 'carer' and 'spouse' roles. 'It's good to be able to talk about it ... [but] I feel selfish ... to turn it and make it about me when I always say to her this is about you'. Matthew's relationship with his wife was transitioning from that of a husband and father to that of a carer. As a couple, he and his wife would share their feelings; as a carer, Matthew did not want his wife, the cancer patient, to feel burdened by his emotions. Thus, managing his own emotions and his wife's emotions was central to his new role.

This new role, as he saw it, was to 'keep on this brave face, to be positive and be a pillar, the father, the head of the house'. He took breaks to sustain himself, but felt guilty doing so. 'I sometimes feel selfish when I am going to see a movie, just to get out of the house, take a break'. He wanted to take on a higher paying position at work, but felt similarly conflicted. 'It would also be a nice pay rise ... But I don't like leaving [her] ... So again I feel selfish'. Talking about his emotions, taking time out for himself, following a job opportunity: these were once reasonable expectations as a husband. Following his wife's diagnosis, roles, priorities and emotional standards changed. His wife's emotional and physical health took primacy: 'I have got to follow her emotions. I have got to follow how she feels. When she has bad days, I have got to be there ... to support'.

This chapter explores spouse cancer carers' role changes and the confusion that this can bring to a spouse's emotions and emotion work. The cancer caregiving

---

1   This chapter is a revised and extended version of the following publication (Olson and Connor, 2014), reproduced here in accordance with the copyright agreement between the first author, Rebecca Olson, and the publisher, Sage: Olson, R.E. and Connor, J. (2014) When They Don't Die: Prognosis Ambiguity, Role Conflict and Emotion Work in Cancer Care. *Journal of Sociology*. http://jos.sagepub.com.ezproxy.uws.edu.au/content/ear ly/2014/08/14/1440783314544996.full.pdf+html.

literature depicts carers' emotional experiences as bifurcated. While many informal carers of cancer patients report high rates of burden, stress, anxiety and unmet needs (Li et al., 2013; Perz et al., 2011), other carers find the caregiving role fulfilling, growing closer to the care recipient (Kramer, 1997; Thompson, 2005). Like this literature, I also found contrasts in carers' stories. In this chapter, I explore one possible impetus behind the variation in carers' emotional experiences: role (un)certainty. In the next chapter I explore another potential explanation.

Some carers in this study were sure of their role(s). These carers described a stronger relationship with their spouse. Others felt frustrated, confused and conflicted about how they should feel. To understand the variations in this role, in this chapter I use theoretical tools from the sociology of emotions to analyse carers' stories of their caregiving journeys with their spouses. Building on Chapter 3, this analysis shows emotion work to be a central feature of the caregiving role, with carers managing their own and their spouse's emotions. With a clearly terminal (negative) prognosis, the role of the spouse cancer carer and the related feeling rules are clear: their spouse's care is their first priority.[2] Though the transition can be difficult, as Matthew's account demonstrates, as time goes on, clear priorities foster more straightforward emotion management and improved social bonds between the carer and spouse with cancer. In contrast, survival past a projected prognosis or a more ambiguous (positive) prognosis – where the cancer patient has a greater chance of survival – can cultivate unclear priorities, role conflict, clashing feeling rules and ongoing feelings of guilt for carers of spouse with cancer.

Before exploring the affects of the patient's prognosis on carers' emotional experiences, this chapter begins with a brief overview of the scholarship on cancer carer burden, allowing for an introduction to the debate in which the analysis took place. The sociology of emotions literature on emotion management and emotional energy is then presented to arm readers with the theoretical tools used in the analysis.[3] Next, the changes in spouses' roles and the emotional and interactionist expectations associated with these roles are examined. Variations in carers' experiences, based in the patient's prognosis are highlighted, demonstrating, perhaps counter-intuitively, the emotional perils of a positive prognosis for carers of a spouse with cancer.

Carer Burden

As noted in the introduction to this book, the onerous nature of family caregiving has been the topic of numerous quantitative studies. This literature shows that carers of cancer patients experience higher rates of stress, anxiety, depression and unaddressed health problems than their non-caregiving counterparts (Burns et al.,

---

2   See Chapter 1 for carers' descriptions of their new priorities and responsibilities.

3   See also Chapter 3 for a brief overview of Hochschild's interactionist theory on emotion work.

2004; Hodges et al., 2005; Northouse et al., 2000; Sharpe et al., 2005; Weitzner et al., 2000). Younger and female caregivers have been found to be more likely to suffer from high rates of burden and unmet needs (Ciambrone and Allen, 2005; Perz et al., 2011; Thomas and Morris, 2002; Ussher and Sandoval, 2008), with female carers least likely to report positive caregiving experiences (Li et al., 2013; Lin et al., 2012).

Specifically, younger carers report knowing less about available services, feeling more burdened by the caregiving role, having more emotional needs and greater unmet needs (Ciambrone and Allen, 2005; Sharpe et al., 2005; Harding and Higginson, 2003; Thomas and Morris, 2002; Burns et al., 2004). Female carers (particularly younger ones) report experiencing higher levels of stress, burden, depression and unmet needs for respite care (Sharpe et al., 2005; Harding and Higginson, 2003; Thomas and Morris, 2002). A subset of carers, however, find caregiving rewarding. Their relationship with the care recipient strengthens, and these carers find satisfaction and purpose in their caregiving role (Mutch, 2010; Williams et al., 2009; Blum and Sherman, 2010; Cassidy, 2013; Kramer, 1997; Thompson, 2005; Weitzner et al., 2000).

The reasons behind these sharp contrasts in carers' perceptions of caregiving are not well understood. Many hypotheses have been proposed for why younger and female carers experience more psychological morbidity and burden, but these hypotheses are at times contradictory. For instance, in a review article on the needs of family cancer carers, Laizner et al. (1993) found that younger carers tend to have greater needs related to coping with their emotions. They suggest that this may be because older carers tend to think of their caring as short term, and therefore cope better. Burns and colleagues (2004: 500), however, suggest that younger working carers have higher rates of unmet needs because 'this group may well have multiple needs and competing role claims' as they juggle family and work responsibilities with their caregiving commitments.[4]

The impetus behind gendered variations in carers' experiences is similarly unclear and contradictory. A range of suggestions for why there are gender differences in carer burden have emerged over the past 30 years. Zarit and colleagues (1986) suggest that differences in caregiver burden may stem from different reporting behaviours, with males under-reporting and females over-reporting psychosocial needs. Pruchno and Resch (1989: 164) suggest that men's needs later in life may be more 'in harmony' with the caregiving role than women of the same age. Braithwaite (1990) suggests that women identify more strongly with the caregiving role, making it more difficult for women to distance themselves emotionally. Two further explanations for women's higher rates of burden related to caregiving are that females spend more time providing care than males and receive less help with caregiving chores (Allen et al., 1999; Northouse et al., 2000). It has been suggested that male carers do fewer caregiver chores,

---

4   Differences in time-sovereignty provide another impetus behind differences in carers' emotional experiences. This thesis is explored in Chapter 5.

receive more help from family and friends with their domestic and caregiving responsibilities and more often rely on formal or paid help for housekeeping and caregiving (Evandrou, 1996; Allen et al., 1999). Other studies, however, have found that men and women provide similar amounts of care and emotional support (Thomas et al., 2001; Ussher and Sandoval, 2008; Perz et al., 2011). Thus, it is still not clear why some carers experience caregiving as fulfilling and others (more often younger and female carers) experience it as burdensome.

In this study, carers' experiences were also divergent – some found the role onerous and others grew closer to their spouse – but age and gender did not account for this variation. To better understand why participants' emotional experiences varied, I again[5] took a sociological approach to analysing carers' emotions, this time using theoretical contributions from Hochschild (1983) and Collins (2004).

Emotion Management and Emotional Energy

As described in Chapter 3, taking an interactionist and sociological approach to understanding the emotions of carers of a spouse with cancer can help us to reimagine emotions as more than internal phenomena or coping responses, but as social, cultural, biological and interpersonal. In this chapter, I use Hochschild's and Collins' theories to further consider the differing social and interactionist aspects of carers' emotional experiences.

Hochschild (1983) argues that manipulation of feelings is central to meeting private and public social expectations. These social expectations, or 'feeling rules', are informed by a complex (and at times contradictory and contested) interplay between social structures, cultural norms, organisational climates and individual roles. Her concept 'emotion work' describes the emotional manipulation that people perform on themselves and others to comply with 'feeling rules' in terms of emotional intensity, direction (positive or negative) and duration in a particular situation (Hochschild, 1983; Turner and Stets, 2005). This emotion work can be shallow or deep. When a person manipulates only their outward display without changing their inner feelings, this is referred to as 'surface acting' (Hochschild, 1983; Wharton, 2009). 'Deep acting' occurs when individuals try to change their inner feelings to comply with feeling rules; when they try to become what is expected of them (Wharton, 2009; Zapf, 2002). If deep acting fails or does not occur, and the emotions a person is required to display on an ongoing basis contradict their inner feelings, 'emotional dissonance' is said to occur leadings to 'a sense of self-estrangement or distress' (Wharton, 2009: 149).

Hochschild's (1983) concept 'emotional labor' refers to the manipulation of one's own emotions to adhere to organisationally defined feeling rules for a wage (Zapf, 2002). A plethora of studies have examined the efforts put into changing one's emotions or feeling displays to adhere to organisational feeling rules.

---

5   See Chapter 3.

These studies have established that emotional labour can contribute to a sense of personal accomplishment or emotional exhaustion, depersonalisation and burnout (Wharton and Erickson, 1995; Zapf, 2002).

Of particular relevance to this analysis is the growing literature on emotional labour in nursing. Huynh et al. (2008), in their systematic review, illustrate the many influences shaping the type of emotional labour undertaken (surface or deep) and outcomes (job satisfaction or burnout). These elements include: organisational norms, job characteristics and identification with one's professional role. Sociologist Deb King (2012), in her research into the emotional labour performed by nurses in aged care facilities, shows that there are two opposing organisational norms or logics of care governing emotions in nursing: bureaucratic models, where efficiency is emphasised, and personalised models, where empathy and emotions take precedence. The former encourages a task, rather than relationship, orientation to care work (King, 2012). The extent to which nurses adhere to these care-emotion logics hinges on a range of factors, including gender and professional socialisation (Huynh et al., 2008).

While 'emotional labour' is a key concept within the sociology of emotions literature, it has been critiqued for being overly rational and negative, and for overlooking agency and authenticity in emotional experiences (King, 2012; Prosser and Olson, 2013). Distinguishing between emotion management at home and at work is another limitation (Wharton and Erickson, 1995). Public and private realms often overlap and commercial relationships are sometimes introduced within private familial life.[6] Privatisation and re-privatisation provide examples of this muddy distinction. Hochschild (2012) examines the emotions of workers and families who outsource 'private' tasks, such as childcare or matchmaking. Emotion work in re-privatised settings – where public work becomes private – has also received attention in Lois' (2006) study of homeschooling mothers. Lois (2006) found that mothers relied on organisationally defined expectations associated with formal classrooms to guide their private emotional labour: schooling their children at home. In doing so, they experienced role strain because teacher-role expectations directly conflicted with the feeling rules associated with their mother role (Lois, 2006). Most mothers eventually burnt out and (re)enrolled their children in school.

Hochschild's theory gives us a language for understanding carers' experiences as at once personal, social, cognitive and embodied. However, it stops short of examining the interaction processes as actors manage their feelings. Collins' (2004) interaction ritual approach makes this process explicit by identifying the ebb and flow of emotional energy that occurs through interaction rituals and is a longer-term emotional tone that an actor experiences in conjunction with others (Collins, 1990; Summers-Effler, 2002). According to Collins' theory, the transfer of positive emotional energy in ritualised interactions can lead to the maintenance

---

6   In Chapter 1, for example, Millicent's story is presented. Millicent used the 'nurse role' to quell her emotions towards her husband's declining health and uncertain prognosis. This strategy is analysed further in a latter portion of Chapter 4.

of micro- (such as interpersonal relationships) and macrostructures (such as religious and national institutions), or it can see an actor's emotional state weaken if the transfer is solely directed in one way or when the actor is required to perform a role that is not authentically emotional to them. Essentially, Collins asserts that maintaining an interaction that feels inauthentic or challenging can cause the actor to feel strain – leading to a diminution of emotional energy. Summers-Effler (2002), furthering Collins' thesis, argues that an actor needs to affirm their self via these rituals and when they cannot, they experience shame, distrust, anxiety and weakened social bonds.

Like Hochschild's work, the explanatory capacity of Collins' theory has also been critiqued. Schwalbe (2007), for example, argues that Collins overemphasises the importance of situated rituals and emotional energy, while underemphasising material and cultural differences. Despite these criticisms, Collins' theory is nonetheless useful to this analysis, offering an additional lens with which to understand emotional exchanges between patient and carer, husband and wife.

Building on the analysis presented in Chapter 3, in this chapter I use Hochschild's concept of emotion work to facilitate discussion of the work that carers of cancer patients do to regulate their own and their spouse's emotions. This emotion work is viewed as part of a person's identity work (Wolkomir, 2001), with felt emotions signifying to oneself and others a person's identity. Following Lois's (2006) examination of the complex emotional labour families perform when a public role becomes private, I also apply labour studies concepts such as role strain and burnout, to understand the emotion work that is performed by carers following deinstitutionalisation (i.e. shifting patient care to the home). Though these labour studies concepts are somewhat limited in their social complexity, they are nonetheless valuable, allowing links to be made across the qualitative analysis presented here and the quantitative conclusions drawn from labour studies research. Collins' work is applied to highlight the need for on-going rituals to create and affirm emotional energy. Through these sociological and labour studies lenses, I find that the prognosis, and the rituals and emotion work done in response to normative expectations surrounding prognoses, provides one explanation for the variation in carers' emotional experiences.

Carers reported that priorities, emotional expectations and relationships changed following the cancer diagnosis, which prompted shifts in their emotional displays and their feelings of guilt. There were, however, important qualitative differences in carers' experiences. Carers of spouses with 'negative' prognoses were able to sustain their new roles, priorities and associated emotion management, and find fulfilment in everyday rituals as a spouse-carer. Carers of spouses with ambiguously 'positive' prognoses were less able to sustain their new roles, describing unclear priorities and contradicting feeling rules associated with being both a spouse and a carer. I start this discussion by presenting the changes to carers' roles and emotion work that accompanied a cancer diagnosis before presenting the contrasts between carers' descriptions of emotion work for a dying spouse and emotion work for a spouse with an unclear prognosis.

Emotion Work for a Newly Diagnosed Spouse

As Matthew's (40s, spouse with breast cancer) story, introduced at the start of this chapter, illustrates, a cancer diagnosis can change and challenge the relationship between husband and wife.[7] The diagnosis prompts a 'readjustment' (Blake, 40s, spouse with breast cancer) within the relationship: a transition to patient and caregiver. Debilitating treatments and the *temporal anomie*[8] that often accompanies a cancer diagnosis bring to the relationship new roles, a new outlook and orientation to the future, and new priorities. Previously interdependent, the cancer diagnosis impelled carers to concentrate on the patient's wellbeing with their own emotions becoming less important. Andrew (60s, spouse with breast cancer) summed these changes up saying, as the carer, 'it's not me that counts'. For Rodney (30s, spouse with breast cancer), caregiving was about:

> Having her [his wife] feel loved and … trying to create the circumstances where she can just focus on herself and not think that she has to worry about me or [our daughter].

In adopting these new priorities, carers performed emotion work to suppress their feeling displays. This involved being 'the strong one … . Even though you are still a little bit jelly' (Jane, 50s, spouse with prostate cancer) or the 'rock' (Sally, 40s, spouse with bladder cancer) for the patient and concealing negative feelings (Anne, 30s, spouse with glandular cancer; Colleen, 60s, spouse with prostate cancer; Fred, 60s, spouse with melanoma; Rodney, 30s, spouse with breast cancer).[9] Sharon (50s, spouse with neurological cancer) worked hard to avoid becoming a 'crying, bawling heap' in front of her husband. Anne explained that:

> At home you try and be brave … because you don't want to cry in front of your child and you have to keep up your strength for your husband because he is the one that is maimed … he is the one coping with all the physical trauma.

Leo (60s, spouse with breast cancer) made a similar evaluation, saying:

> Much as … carers … will probably feel sorry for themselves, thinking, "Why me? Why should it happen?" … their predicament isn't still as bad as [the patient] – facing pain, premature death and perhaps not fulfilling ambition[s] … grandchildren and this and that.

---

7 See Chapter 1 for an analysis of the cancer diagnosis of as the introduction of a new 'figured world' into a marriage.

8 See Chapter 3.

9 Like Thomas et al.'s (2002: 538) study, this research found that both female and male carers concealed their own emotions for what they saw as their spouse's benefit.

These two expectations – that the carer suppress their emotions and simultaneously provide emotional support to the patient – made the emotion work associated with caregiving particularly onerous. This ongoing emotion management and maintenance of a brave face was very tiring, because 'you are not allowed to be weak' (Sally, 40s, spouse with bladder cancer). Helping the patient to manage their emotions meant that the carer also had to manage their own emotions. Carers, however, received very little emotional support and had few outlets when the focus of their emotion management was their spouse, the very person they would normally turn to for support. In Fred's (60s, spouse with melanoma) assessment, based in his experience as a patient and a carer, 'The supporter is definitely a harder thing, because for us I was trying to support [my wife] and keep myself afloat'.

Lapses were a source of guilt. Ian (50s, spouse with breast cancer), who was introduced at the start of the book, recounted his remorse at his wife's disappointment when he was not able to suppress his emotions and provide her with support. My wife 'feels that … that I wasn't encouraging enough. Obviously, it leaked all out, that I … sort of saw her dead'. Charlie (50s, spouse with breast cancer) confessed that 'we still have the odd blow up occasionally where it gets to you, and you think, "Oh shit, I shouldn't have done that"'. When he feels the need to 'blow off a bit of steam' he goes to the pub, but finds 'I feel guilty about it sometimes' for prioritising his own emotions and for leaving her by herself, fearful that she might need his support while he is away. Andrew (60s, spouse with breast cancer) similarly found that 'there are times when you get a little bit upset …. When I do get frustrated', but this causes him to feel 'a bit guilty – you remember that this [cancer] is ongoing'.

Following the cancer diagnosis, spouse carers both struggled to and succeeded in concealing their emotions. They performed surface acting emotion work to display the varying facades expected of them as supportive spouses. All participants described changes in priorities, roles and feeling rules following their spouses' cancer diagnosis that prompted this emotion work. However, as the months dedicated to caregiving marched on, those caring for a spouse with an imminent terminal prognosis were able to sustain these new priorities, gaining a sense of accomplishment from sharing time and emotional energy with their spouse, and fulfilling their spouse-carer role. Those caring for a spouse with an ambiguous prognosis were not as successful in sustaining the priorities associated with cancer caregiving and, instead of fulfilment, described guilt and confusion associated with contradictory feeling rules and roles.

Emotion Work for a Dying Spouse

Bernard, Judy and Fred were caring for spouses with short terminal prognoses, where their spouses were told it was unlikely that they would survive more than a certain number of months. Bernard (50s) recalled their subsequent shift in priorities, focus, feeling rules and closeness. His wife was diagnosed with metastatic breast cancer nine months before our first interview. She died one month before our interview. Since her diagnosis, 'It was a single focus' – his wife. In addition to managing her pain and care, Bernard worked to keep his wife's spirits lifted:

> At times [my wife] would say, 'oh I am a burden. You need to get on with life' … I would say, 'hang on, we don't use that word around here', and 'you have carried me for most of the journey'.

> You just have to forget the bad things. You try and actually put those out of mind and focus on the good things … nice flowers … a lovely call from someone … I needed to be 'there' because what would you do to a loved one if you were so negative?[10]

Bernard was 'absolutely run ragged' managing his wife's emotions and care. He suffered from depression and anxiety that led to irritable bowel syndrome. Despite his illness, he rarely took breaks. He did not leave her side unless someone was there with his wife. A counsellor advised him to 'take a bit of space, go for a walk … slow down a bit'. But, he objected saying, 'That is easy to say, difficult to do … It was easier to stay on the treadmill than it was to [get off], because there was a certain sense of guilt if you even took time out'. Yet, Bernard found that this change in their relationship, feeling rules and priorities ironically made their relationship stronger at the end of his wife's life.

> You get, you probably get a lot closer to a partner than in a normal course of life … it [cancer] brought us so much closer …. It's part of life's experience isn't it (crying).

Three months before our first interview, Judy's (60s) husband was diagnosed with an asbestos-related cancer with poor survival rates. Before his diagnosis, she was retired but working part time. After the diagnosis, she focused solely on caregiving, because 'it's what you do when you get married'. Their relationship and interactions changed as a result of his waning health. 'This is a man who has always been self-reliant … physically leaning on me, crying, saying, "I don't know what to do"'. He was more dependent on her and more appreciative of her. 'He hasn't criticised a meal for a very long time'. They were also 'as a couple … much closer'.

> We are like a pair of silly old idiots. We go for a walk in the evening holding hands. We never used to do that …. We [sit] out in the dark on the veranda and we [talk] about the past … it [is] just lovely.

---

10 See Chapter 3 for a full elaboration on Bernard's 'positive but realistic' approach to emotion work and caregiving.

Although their rituals as a married couple strengthened their bond, Judy was careful to balance her caregiving and marital role. She had witnessed the way relationships can change when a spouse is highly dependent for a long period of time.

> I worry that I get too bossy … that I will turn into one of those terrible people who dominates … . Why should you in your last years start feeling like you are a waste of space? (crying).

She reflected on her interactions with her husband to prevent this from happening. 'The last thing I wanted was for him to feel stupid, useless, a nuisance … . So part of my job is to keep him feeling significant'. Ironically, to ensure that her husband felt significant, she occasionally got short with him.

> I sometimes snap at him, but … I think that I would do that when he was at his best … I mean, if I gave into him on every single thing, that would be sort of indicating … I don't respect you … I am just going along with you. It's patronising … I am running this fine line between trying not to be patronising and trying not to be dominating.

Their disagreement about cooking utensils offers an example of how Judy used arguments to help her husband feel independent.

> I stirred him up the other day … it was quite deliberate because frankly I was getting a bit sick of him being so nice … (laughter). No. I mean he is a nice person, but we are not always lovely dovey. And I had bought him this eighty-four dollar saucepan … because he always cooks his own porridge … . I bought him this special plastic spoon too and he won't use it. Anyway, this morning the sound of that metal spoon was irritating me so much … . I pushed him and I said, 'For god sake, you say you won't use the plastic spoon because you will end up eating plastic. You are scraping all the Teflon off the bottom. You are going to be eating that!' And he flew back and said, 'Oh, you think you know everything' or something. And I said, 'Bravo love. Good on you'. And he said, 'What are you talking about?' And I said, 'I wanted to see if you were still your old self'. He gave me this look.

Overall, her husband's dependence and caregiving demands changed their emotional expectations and roles, but Judy actively managed their interactions, successfully balancing feeling rules. The result was enhanced closeness.

Fred's (60s) wife was diagnosed with secondary melanoma and given a six-month prognosis. This substantially changed their relationship.

> From that point [the diagnosis] … Jane became my prime focus … . When we got married, we looked at the words in our ceremony and … we tried to [say]

that we would allow each other to grow in our own way without stopping each other …. But once Jane was [diagnosed] … this made my focus more Jane … my role was to be her support.

With this changed focus came emotion work. As the husband-carer, Fred tried to be the hopeful, selfless companion: 'I was trying to support Jane and keep myself afloat'. Slip ups prompted remorse.

> Jane said to me, 'What are you thinking?' I said, 'Well I am thinking what I am going to say at your funeral and I feel guilty about that. I feel like I am being unfaithful to you'.

As part of his new priorities and emotional project of lifting his wife's spirits, Fred and Jane went travelling to places Jane wanted to go. 'We took off four months, [went] over to Perth … Darwin … I wanted to do these things for her … I wasn't sure she was going to be around in six months'. But, as Jane lived more than seven months past her diagnosis, Fred started to feel 'resentment'.

> I got tired of doing everything for Jane and … I started to feel guilty …. Something would happen and I would say, 'Geez I don't want to do this! Oh Jane mightn't be around so I will do that'. Then I started to feel … uncomfortable and then I would feel guilty about that …. A word that you could use around the six, seven, eight, nine months, was … resentment. 'What are you still doing here?' And that sounds really nasty, but I had been focused on this six months … and she is still around. It's seven months and I am happy about that, but I am thinking hang on, maybe I can ease off on this now. Maybe I can do the things that I want.

Five years after her six-month prognosis,[11] Jane was still alive and their old priorities returned. Despite Fred's feelings of discomfort, guilt and resentment, he said that cancer had 'drawn us together'.

For carers of a dying spouse, the feeling rules, roles and identity work were onerous, but clear. These caregivers prioritised caring for their spouses, worked on improving their spouses' 'spirits' and consequently described strengthened social bonds as couples.[12] For carers of a spouse whose cancer was not in the terminal stage, as Fred's extended experience illustrates, the emotion work was confusing for two reasons: the uncertain boundary between carer and spouse, and the ambiguous nature of the patient's future.

---

11   As discussed in Chapter 2.

12   In Leo's (60s, spouse with breast cancer) assessment, 'we are closer together the last few years, emotionally, psychologically, because problems always bring people closer together, like war'.

Emotion Work for a Spouse with an Ambiguous Prognosis

Spouses entered into roles as caregiver and patient, but they were still married couples. During times of intense caregiving the required balance was clear. But, if the patient's health improved and months or years devoted to caring were extended, the imbalance between being a carer and spouse became more tiring and fraught with guilt. When the illness trajectory was uncertain, carers were not sure when their role ended. They wondered, 'Will it ever end? ... Will our relationship ever be the same again?' (Fiona, 60s, spouse with prostate cancer). They felt they could not sustain these roles indefinitely, but in turn felt guilt for wanting to give their own emotions and lives precedence. Millicent's and Linda's stories typify this experience.

Millicent's (60s, spouse haematological cancer) emotion management involved an inward struggle. After caregiving for 16 years, in the months before our first interview she could see that he was struggling with his loss of independence. 'He has become quite frail just in the last couple of months ... he is feeling that he is losing his control and power .... He finds that hard'. His increasing frailty meant he relied more heavily on Millicent for his mobility and physical support. Millicent grew 'resentful' of rising repeatedly in the night to help her husband to the toilet and became 'sick of having to do everything'. But, she said, 'It is difficult to know how to handle it'.

She sometimes lashed out at him when they disagreed, but then felt immediate remorse.

> Sometimes I would get really short with him and almost be cruel .... He has this special chair ... it was sort of a tippy tilty chair. And he was comfortable for a little while and then he felt he wanted to sit up. And I said, 'If I sit the chair forward, you are going to fall out'. He said, 'But I want to stand up. I want to stand up'. I said, 'Alright then'. And I just tipped it up and he nearly fell out of the chair. See? And then, I felt terrible because his eyes looked really hurt. I thought, 'Oh, how awful I have been'. I was angry .... I said, 'I am so sorry. I am so sorry' .... So I had moments of anger and then I felt real guilt about those times. I thought, 'How could I be so mean?'

Overall, her response was to withdraw: it was easier to approach caring as an emotionally detached formal carer or nurse because this allowed her to shield her emotions and 'stay in control'.[13] But, she felt unsure about playing the nurse instead of the wife role and sought reassurance asking me, 'I don't know if that happens with everyone or whether it is just me. Have you found this in your talks with people?' Later on in the interview she assessed her emotion management approach as inappropriate.

---

13   See Chapter 1.

> When he gets a little bit, almost weepy, I tend to get more … matter of fact (crying) … . I don't get myself too involved in that yet … I don't want us both to break down. But yet we are going to have to do that, we are going to have to weep together sometime … . I think I am really handling it the wrong way, but I guess in the ideal world I would be seeing a counsellor or a social worker or something like that and saying how should I be doing this as a good wife? … . I am probably doing a lot of things wrong.

Millicent's requests for advice illustrate the emotional uncertainty and guilt that caregivers feel when their spouse's trajectory is uncertain.

Linda's (40s) story provides further insight into the hazy boundary between being a spouse and carer, and the correspondingly complex emotion management. Although her husband was diagnosed with a terminal bowel cancer, he underwent radical surgery and, at the time of our second interview, improved so much that he was working again, part-time. When he was initially unwell, the feeling rules and priorities were obvious.

> When I have been intensively caring, I haven't had time to think about it really, about how I am actually feeling. So, I hadn't actually – there hasn't been time for the uncertainty, it was … so intensive … . In terms of me needing to be a full on carer, the emotional side was easier to cope with because it was actually about survival and he was just trying to survive and I was doing all the giving and he was doing all the taking.

As her husband's wellbeing improved, her emotion management priorities became unclear, particularly about how to respond when he was 'horrible' to her.

> It gets to a point where you start having to wind back a bit as they are getting better and let them do things for themselves and they may have frustrations … he could do things, couldn't do some things … . I did manage to ease off, then my role is then becoming more of a mixture of wife and carer, so that is where the complexity starts to come in … you can be too ill to have the situation where you are lashing out, because … you don't have the energy … you are too busy trying to survive. Then you get to a point where … you are actually well enough to be awful to your carer.

When he was in remission, he was on a three-monthly scan cycle to check for recurrences. The scans caused him severe anxiety and to 'lash out' temporarily at her. Linda was angry and confused.

> The uncertainty I feel is about feeling guilty about feeling really angry with him … I think, 'should I be behaving totally as if he has never been sick and he is just fine' … saying, 'Look, just cut that out'. And yet you know that the driver behind that is precisely because he has been through this process … I am a bit at sea …

because it's complex; it's tied up in a marriage as well as tied up in a caregiver. That's where I am uncertain, between the carer and the wife side. And how to then respond .... Is this about being a carer or is this about being a wife? Am I being unfair? Am I not tapping in well enough to the whole huge emotional, psychological toll this has had on him? .... What does that do to a marriage?

Linda had been discussing her difficulties with a cancer support group and planned to seek advice from a marriage counsellor.

As time went on for those patients outside of the terminal stage and they became well enough to exhibit irritating idiosyncrasies and express criticisms, carers became exasperated. Spouse-appropriate feelings of resentment and anger were often followed by shame for not maintaining carer-appropriate feelings of tolerance. Crucially, carer and spouse feeling rules were at odds. As Linda explained, it would be acceptable for her, as a wife, to feel anger towards her husband (and act on it), but if a carer were to feel and act the same way, it would be construed as 'bullying'. Conversely, if a patient were cruel to a carer, a carer would be expected to see these insults as a result of the patient's frustration and refrain from feeling upset. However, if a spouse were to hold back from responding to an insult, they would be viewed as a 'doormat'.[14] Herein lies the emotion management difficulty and self-prioritisation complication: the ambiguity of the carer role parameters.

Like those caring for a dying spouse, Millicent and Linda engaged in deep acting emotion work. But, because their husbands' prognoses were not clear, prioritisation of their conflicting feeling rules as wife and carer was confusing. Using labour studies terminology, Millicent and Linda's experiences would be described as role conflict, where contradictory goals and job requirements cause 'uncertainty in how to proceed' (Zapf, 2002: 253). Thus, instead of experiencing the enhanced closeness and improved solidarity described by carers of a dying spouse, these participants described confusion, unclear feeling rules and feelings of guilt.

Emotional Dissonance

One carers' experience of contradictory feeling rules was so extreme that it caused 'emotional dissonance'. Phyllis (50s), introduced in Chapter 1, cared for her husband whose neurological cancer caused his personality to change and memory to atrophy. After the onset of symptoms she described him as 'a bit like a two year old'. The changes to his cognitive abilities and personality were so great that their emotional relationship ended with the onset of his symptoms. Phyllis tried to organise activities

---

14   Judy used similar language in elaborating on the importance of arguing to her strategy of helping her husband to feel important. 'Any couple will argue .... If you don't stand your ground over something you think is right, then what are you? A doormat?'

such as picnics or trips to the cinema to enjoy the time left with her husband, but found her husband no longer cared if they shared experiences together.

Phyllis felt trapped. She wanted her husband to die so that she could be released from the role. Although these sentiments might be socially acceptable as a formal carer, they are not socially acceptable as a wife. Phyllis managed her feelings on the surface, pretending to all but her closest friends and family that she was hopeful of a cure and wanting her husband to live as long as possible. As described in Chapter 1, Phyllis 'put on this big act' for extended family and medical professionals when test results came back showing the tumour had not grown.[15]

In our second interview, she elaborated on her emotion work, saying she would avoid answering the phone to avoid having to pretend.

> I wouldn't answer the phone because people would ask what happened with the MRI and I thought, 'I can't go through it again. I can't' ... . I couldn't face telling these [people] and putting it on ... . I was really draining because you thought, 'I don't like lying to people'. You feel really dishonest and then you feel guilty for feeling that way yourself. So it brings up all these other emotions ... It's really hard ... . A lot of people haven't got any idea what it's like to be going through it. They don't see how difficult it is. What we are expected to do. The social norms. We are expected to do this, feel that or the other. It's difficult.

For Phyllis, the priorities, roles and emotion work expected of her were clear: she was to selflessly prioritise caring for her husband, raising his emotional state and helping him to find meaning in their final months together. However, the lack of reciprocity, her husband's changed personality and their lack of meaningful interaction left Phyllis unable to alter her emotions to match social expectations. This illustrates the centrality of meaningful interactions to emotion management.

Prognoses, Feeling Rules and Emotional Energy

This inductive analysis of carers of cancer patients' experiences, underpinned by Hochschild's and Collins' theories, presents one possible explanation for variation in perceptions of caregiving. While priorities, feeling norms and family roles change with a cancer diagnosis, the certainty and value (positive or negative) of the prognosis and the capacity of the patient to share in reciprocated rituals shapes spouse-carers' emotions. Terminal prognoses facilitated clear priorities, emotion management and improved social bonds; ambiguous 'positive' prognoses fostered role conflict, contradictory feeling rules and ongoing guilt. Counter-intuitively, the certainty of death makes it easier for spouse carers to manage their emotions.

---

15   See Chapters 1 and 2 for a more in-depth overview of Phyllis's caregiving experience.

After a spouse's cancer diagnosis, carers have a particular identity position to fulfil within the family interaction ritual (Collins, 2004), which requires them to perform surface acting (Hochschild, 1983) and present a positive emotional 'face' to family, friends and the patient, irrespective of their own feelings. This surface acting has been linked with emotional exhaustion and burnout in labour studies (Wharton, 2009). Family carers, however, are expected to suppress their emotions and desires, and maintain a supportive facade. Veering from these expectations prompts feelings of guilt.

For carers of a dying spouse, ongoing spouse-carer emotion work is sustained by new priorities of facilitating emotional-energy rich rituals with one's spouse that prompt improved solidarity between husband and wife and a sense of accomplishment – what is referred to as 'living in the now' in Chapter 3. These carers suspended other roles to prioritise spending time with their dying spouse. In doing so, they gained positive emotional energies (pride and fulfilment), which strengthened their micro-interaction ritual investment in their role and marriage. Spouse-carer identity fulfilling and reciprocated positive emotional energies (Collins, 1990) resulted when the emotions that caregivers' experienced (after interactional emotion work) matched those expected of them. In labour studies, a perceived balance between emotional investments and returns prevents feelings of emotional exhaustion, depersonalisation and reduced accomplishment (Lois, 2006; Zapf, 2002), lending support to this finding. Sensing and expressing positive emotions, because of deep emotion work, has also been linked with feelings of accomplishment and job satisfaction (Wharton, 2009; Zapf, 2002).

When positive emotional energy is not reciprocated, as was the case for one couple in this study (Phyllis and her husband), there is a perceived imbalance in emotional investment, which may lead to emotional exhaustion and emotional dissonance. Emotional interactions are reciprocal. When the interaction lacks passion (even negative), the interaction can be deeply disturbing for the initiator – leading to a void of emotions and a decreased desire for interaction. The role conflict arising from normative social expectations of hoping for 'good' test results versus the reality of wishing it was 'over', deeply challenges the emotional state and ability of carers to engage with their spouse and wider social networks. Compounding this is a carer's reduced time sovereignty,[16] preventing them from engaging in other social opportunities. Labour studies show that emotional exhaustion (a precursor to burnout) is exacerbated by depersonalisation. When emotional exhaustion occurs, people may take part in depersonalisation, receding from emotional involvement and decreasing further their sense of accomplishment (Lois, 2006). In the example provided in this study, depersonalisation was imposed upon the carer by her husband's disease. Depersonalised interactions prevented Phyllis from achieving a sense of accomplishment in her work as a carer, leaving her emotionally exhausted and at risk of burnout. Using Collins' (1990) theory, I might similarly suggest that imposed depersonalisation, because of disease or

---

16   See the Introduction and Chapter 5.

another cause, puts marriages at risk as the positive emotional energy required to sustain these social bonds is deficient.[17]

For carers of a spouse with a more 'positive' prognosis, spouse-carer emotion work was undermined by ambiguous priorities, leaving carers unsure of which roles and feeling rules they should follow: those for spouses or carers. Contradictory feeling rules have been linked to burnout in labour studies (Zapf, 2002). Burnout has been linked to poor health, including 'psychosomatic complaints, depression, and other long-term stress effects' (Zapf, 2002: 256). Role conflict has also been found to be a strong predictor of burnout (Lee and Ashforth, 1996; Lois, 2006; Zapf, 2002). One carer, Millicent, tried to overcome her role conflict by prioritising task-oriented formal carer (nurse) feeling rules and withdrawing (depersonalisation) from her husband (see King, 2012), but found this difficult because of the guilt she felt for not being a 'good wife'. Lois (2006) made a similar finding about homeschooling mothers: depersonalisation was not an option because mothers could not emotionally withdraw from their relationship with their child and see themselves as 'good mothers'. Lois (2006) suggests that this is because who we are defines how we feel about a situation and vice versa (Hochschild, 1983). Being a 'good' mother or spouse is often central to core identities, and thus difficult to change (Wolkomir, 2001).

Conclusion

With patient care increasingly outsourced from institutions to families the meaning and emotional experiences of cancer for patients and families is changing. Advances in treatment continue to improve survival rates, but simultaneously increase the number of ambiguous 'positive' prognoses. In seeking to understand carers' differing journeys and improve support for these carers shouldering the weight of these changes, it is imperative that we examine the social and interactional characteristics of carers' experiences. This will serve to better prepare health professionals as they screen carers for psychological morbidity and support them in their roles (Given et al., 2012; Given et al., 2006).

The findings presented in this chapter provide one alternative hypothesis to understanding carers' varying experiences of caregiving as rewarding or burdensome, supported by theories from the sociology of emotions and findings from labour studies research. Clear priorities and feeling rules, and shared positive emotional-energy rituals may be central to understanding why some carers, those caring for a spouse with a terminal cancer, experience caregiving as rewarding. In contrast, the role conflict and contradictory feeling rules associated with ambiguous 'positive' prognoses potentially explains why other carers have high rates of stress and burden. In Chapter 5, I present another hypothesis for understanding carers diverging experiences of caregiving: differences in time-sovereignty.

---

17   A number of carers recounted incidents of celebrities and friends who left their spouses following a cancer diagnosis.

Chapter 5

Time: A Time-Sovereignty Approach to Understanding Carers' Emotions and Support Preferences[1]

I was surprised when Joe described phone calls from friends as 'bothersome'. Joe (60s, spouse with ovarian cancer) had what might be described as an onerous caregiving role. His wife died a couple years before our first interview. He had been her carer intermittently throughout the preceding 20 years during times of treatment and recovery. He took an active role in supporting her emotionally when she was unwell and continued to support her as a husband during remission. In her final year, her mobility declined because of a metastasis to her brain. Thus, Joe supported her in completing activities of daily living, such as showering, toileting and dressing her, in addition to continuing to provide emotional and practical support. About phone calls, he said:

> The phone didn't stop ringing ... people would get home from work and at about six o'clock the phone would start .... I eventually had to take the phone off the hook so I had time to prepare a meal.

Answering numerous calls made it difficult for him to complete caring tasks that needed to be accomplished, so he avoided the phone and sent mass emails to family and friends instead.

> I set up an email group list and there were a couple of [my wife's] very close friends that we said you can call in or you can phone, but I asked everyone else not to phone, that I would send out regular updates. I used to send out a weekly bulletin and various people heard and asked to be put on that group list. We had a circulation of about 84 in the end.

---

1   This chapter is a modified and expanded version of the following publication (Olson, 2014b), which has been reused here in accordance with the copyright agreement between the author, Rebecca Olson, and the publisher, John Wiley & Sons Ltd: Olson, R.E. (2014b) A Time-Sovereignty Approach to Understanding Carers of Cancer Patients' Experiences and Support Preferences. *European Journal of Cancer Care* 23, 239–48. Doi: 10.1111/ecc.12121 http://onlinelibrary.wiley.com/doi/10.1111/ecc.12121/abstract.

Joe was not alone in describing phone calls from friends as a nuisance. Fiona (60s, spouse with prostate cancer) described phone calls as 'tiresome'.

> You would come home at night and then ... people mean well I know, but there's three million messages on the phone all wanting to know is everything fine and you think, 'oh god, I can't make one more phone call'. ... You sort of get a bit swamped with people meaning well. So I found that a bit ... tiresome on a daily basis ... . It was just all a bit onerous at the time.

Sally (40s, spouse with bladder cancer) also saw the phone as a 'burden' and a disruption from caring:

> The telephone does become quite a burden almost and then people call and they want to talk and be supportive, and that's really really nice, but wow, you know, there are quite a few of them.

Others carers, however, were glad to have the interruption and distraction that phone calls provided. Andrew (60s, spouse with breast cancer) viewed phone calls as a welcome diversion from his anxiety and distress. Carl (70s, spouse with lung cancer) called it a vital source of 'moral support ... . They just phone up and have long conversations'. Laughing or discussing someone else's life provided these carers with a break from focusing on cancer. These carers described telephone conversations as an essential line to inclusion and emotional support. Mary (50s, spouse with prostate cancer), for instance, explained that phone calls are a means of engaging in more intimate and longer conversations than those she had in person. She concluded, 'the phone is a wonderful mechanism'. She even called the emotional support she received over the telephone a 'need'.

> There is one friend in particular ... she will make a point of phoning at least every four weeks. And she will always make a point of ... asking how I am dealing with it ... which is really lovely ... . My need is to be able to talk about it to people, and to have people whom I trust enough ... and like enough, to be able to talk to them.

Judy (60s, spouse with asbestos-related cancer) described talking to friends and family as an essential opportunity to release and offload, saying 'bawl[ing] [her] eyes out' to her sister over the phone was a helpful release. For two other carers, telephone conversations about emotions and experiences were described as a 'useful' and unobtrusive method of requesting support. Venting to friends and family made others aware of the carer's troubles and often prompted the listener to offer practical or emotional support.

These contrasts in carers' perceptions of phone calls caught my interest, prompting me to ask, 'Why was the phone perceived in such black and white extremes by so many carers?' While this could just be a matter of individual preference, as discussed in the previous chapter, the literature on carers' experiences suggests that their experiences vary by age and gender. Younger carers report higher rates of burden and unmet needs and less awareness of services (Thomas and Morris, 2002; Harding and Higginson, 2003; Burns et al., 2004; Ciambrone and Allen, 2005). Older carers are more likely to experience a benefit of caregiving: growing closer to the care-recipient (Grbich et al., 2001; McNamara, 2001; Thomas et al., 2002; Thompson, 2005). Female carers report higher levels of stress, burden, depression and unmet needs for respite care than male carers (Sharpe et al., 2005; Ussher and Sandoval, 2008; Perz et al., 2011). However, neither gender nor age provided any clarity. Husbands and wives were equally represented among both those who appreciated telephone calls and those who found them burdensome, as were carers in their 40s, 50s and 60s.

Examining the temporal aspects of carers' experiences did provide more clarity, offering another possible reason behind the poorly understood variations in carers' emotional experiences. Building on the analysis presented in Chapter 4, in this chapter, I explore time-sovereignty, or the extent to which carers' had control over their time, as another means of understanding divergences in carers' experiences.

Time-sovereignty, it will be shown here, also provides possible answers to another question to emerge from the cancer caregiving literature: why do perceptions of support services differ across carers? Little is known about the value of support services for carers of cancer patients. Research with cancer patients shows attending support groups decreases distress and depression, and improves role adjustment and coping (Docherty, 2004; Herron, 2005; Pearson, 2006). Individual therapy has been found to improve stress, anxiety, depression, mood and overall psychological morbidity in patients (Boudioni et al., 2000; Boulton et al., 2001; Pearson, 2006).

Research on the value of support services for cancer carers is limited. Many studies examine their efficacy generally; few identify how they are helpful to carers of cancer patients specifically (Pearson, 2006). Research on the value of support services to informal carers of patients with many diagnoses provides further insight and questions. Counselling has been found to reduce carer burden and depression, improve wellbeing and legitimise the importance of carers' emotions (Boulton et al., 2001; Sörensen et al., 2002). Face-to-face support groups help carers to continue caring and facilitate information sharing, on the disease and emotions (Sörensen et al., 2002; Chambers et al., 2001; Harding and Higginson, 2003). Respite services decrease carer depression and improve wellness (Sörensen et al., 2002), but only 8 per cent of Australian carers in need of respite access it (Gibson et al., 1996). Government financial support is available to Australian carers, but it is unclear how payments help and why a mere 15 per cent of carers access them (Hughes, 2007). Furthermore, few studies examine why support preferences vary (Weitzner et al., 2000; Boulton et al., 2001; Thomas and Morris, 2002; Pearson, 2006).

In this chapter, I examine the variation in carers' emotional experiences and support preferences. Analysis, using a theoretical framework based on 'discretionary time', shows that carers with few competing commitments and less demanding caregiving responsibilities had time to experience and unpack the range of emotions associated with cancer, and reconnect with their spouse. These carers preferred emotion-focused support. In contrast, carers with multiple commitments had little time to themselves and viewed emotions as an indulgence they could little afford. These carers preferred practical support.

I start by illustrating the temporal variations in carers' experiences by relaying five carers' stories. I then use the literature on discretionary time to map carers' temporal experiences onto two continuums: one related to the temporal nature of their caregiving responsibilities and the other related to the other demands on their time. This schema is then applied to an analysis of carers' varied emotional experiences and support preferences.

Time to Care

Fred and Jane, Joe, Anne and Sally – their stories show that time is clearly a central factor in understanding the range in carers' emotional experiences and needs. Carers' experiences varied depending not just on how much time they spent caring, but on how much control they had over their time. Some care work was mildly demanding. For others it was extremely demanding of their time and energy. Others still were giving care to more than one person in addition to fulfilling their paid employment and childrearing responsibilities, leaving them with little control over their time.

Fred and Jane

Fred and Jane, the couple in their 60s introduced in Chapter 2, took turns as carers and patients. First Jane was diagnosed with melanoma. A few years later, Fred was diagnosed with prostate cancer. Despite the calls on their time from caregiving, they generally had control over their time. They were retired from full-time work, their children were grown and their cancers and treatment were not physically debilitating. Thus, they had time to experience and interpret their emotions.

Of the emotional side of cancer, Jane said 'it actually brought us really close'. But, it was a lot of work. 'He had a really bad time … for a long time', so trying to lift his spirits was 'constant'. Jane said this was difficult because she was not sure how to go about doing this.

Fred struggled with feelings of guilt, fear and uncertainty as a husband and a carer when his wife was diagnosed. 'I know that it's ridiculous. I felt that I had failed her family because she was in good health when I married her … and I really felt the pending loss'. But, they talked to each other and cancer support groups and they learned to manage their emotions. They distracted themselves with a trip around Australia on their motorbike. They learned ways of overcoming sleepless nights. As a result, Fred assessed their relationship to be 'stronger'.

Joe

Joe (60s) retired when his wife became disabled and fully dependent on him for care as a result of metastatic ovarian cancer. They had no children. Joe alone took on the cooking, cleaning and communicating with family and friends, taking only a few hours respite care each week to do the grocery shopping and run errands. He would wake up when his wife stirred at night to turn her in bed because she was no longer able to roll over herself. This left him sleep deprived, but he said the experience had brought them closer together.

> My wife had some very radical treatment at the time … and I think that experience pulled us closer together …. I think it brought us closer together and made us realise our own mortality.

He cried telling me how much it meant to hug her. He said, 'she was in the later stage of the disease …. Just to be able to lie together and hug each other was, I think (crying) that was probably important for [my wife] too'. When I asked him what his biggest needs were, he replied:

> My biggest need was more time …. Just more time to do everything that had to be done. It was a pretty full-time thing. I was existing on two or three hours' sleep I think. So, it was just a very demanding period.

Clearly, with Joe existing on little sleep and caring day and night for his wife, he was time-poor. Yet, he did have enough time to experience the benefits of caregiving: growing emotionally closer with his wife.

Anne

Anne (30s) is the mother of a toddler, a receptionist and was caring for her husband who had a rare glandular cancer. Since his diagnosis, disfiguring surgery and radiation treatment, Anne had become the breadwinner in addition to her other responsibilities. This meant that Anne worked six days a week.

Anne described herself as physically and emotionally exhausted. She cried throughout the first interview and said she was drinking more at night to cope with her lack of control over her life. Anne did not say that the cancer experience brought her closer to her husband. Instead, her emotions were saturated with guilt related to her lack of time. She said:

> Time is the biggest need …. There are days when I feel like I am cracking up and I think I can't keep doing this. I cannot keep up this pace …. It seems everything I do, I feel guilty. If I am taking a time out at the gym, or playing with my daughter then I am not earning money. But even if I am earning money I feel guilty because you know, money, guilt, time. It's my little horrible triangle.

Sally

Sally (40s) is another carer and a mother of three teenage daughters. In addition to caring for her husband who was diagnosed with bladder cancer and was undergoing surgery and radiation therapy, she was also a carer for two elderly parents and worked (in paid employment) part-time. She is a clear example of a woman in the sandwich generation: caring for her parents and in-laws, her children and her husband. She used the analogy of a snowball for her caregiving. She said:

> I have had rapid deterioration in health and the death of my father and deterioration of health of my mother, and my father-in-law all happening over the last two years. It's sort of like a snowball … one that just seems to keep getting a bit larger, and I am aware of a sense in myself that I am pretty sick of it (laughs) … . Just so much looking after people to do.

Using meiosis, she said caregiving leaves her feeling less than 'refreshed'.

> Always sort of rushing off to take somebody who is very old to the dentist or get their prescriptions or every time you get home there are two or three messages … you don't know whether it's a drama or whether it's not a crisis that you need to resolve for one of them … . When I go down and see either of the older people, I usually come back a little bit tight lipped and stressed in some way. Yeah, because my mother has lots of … demands … . I leave with a long list of things I need to get her and bring her and do for her that she has asked. And, for the father-in-law who has dementia, it's a different sort of stress of sort of wondering whether he is really being looked after well enough. Just seeing someone always having wet trousers and that sort of thing is just, yeah. So you tend to get home not refreshed.

During her husband's time in hospital, she felt angry towards him for continuing to smoke after the doctor advised him to quit. Since that time, though, she has put her emotions aside. She says she sees her feelings as an indulgence for which she does not have time.

> Sally: I didn't really go work through emotional things … . It is partly that, I am a little bit scared what you will find. And then if it doesn't work out, the way I saw my job was to look after [my husband] and three other girls [and] two older parents. If you delve into the emotional and it doesn't resolve in a way, then you are in a mess, then what is going to happen? So … keep that gate closed (laughs).
>
> R: So maybe because you knew so many people were counting on you, you couldn't … indulge yourself …

Sally: That is exactly the word I was thinking. I do think of it that way. And I don't think it's necessarily the right way to think about it.

[Later on in the interview]

Sally: There is a shortage of it, that is the greatest issue with time. So, in terms of things like even then, how you deal with the emotional things, there is really no time for it. There really aren't enough hours in the day with all those things happening.

With so many people relying on her, Sally did not have time to feel. She did, however, *need* time to digest and emotionally respond to information about her husband's cancer.

That processing takes quite a while, especially when they are big nasty bits of information. Isn't that funny how ... I have to run over it and run over it (laughs) to actually absorb it somehow.

Time and Social Welfare

It is clear from these narratives that time was significant in shaping carers' emotional experiences. To understand why time was so significant, I turned to the sociological theories of time as an empirical measurement of social welfare. As Szollos (2009: 336) explains 'time shortage and being rushed clearly interfere with quality of life. Conversely, time affluence and some unencumbered free time would likely enhance the quality of life'. Goodin and colleagues' (2008) concept of 'discretionary time', and its underlying theoretical framework, provides a useful tool for understanding why some carers' experiences are time-pressured. Discretionary time is defined as 'time which is free to spend as one pleases' (Goodin et al., 2008: i). Others have used similar terms like 'time sovereignty' to denote a person's freedom to control their working time schedule and when to do certain tasks within their work days (see Davies, 2001: 136; Roberts, 2002: 176). In contrast, Goodin et al.'s focus is not solely on work time, but on the autonomy one has over time in all life domains.

Discretionary time incorporates each person's (culturally grounded) commitments and basic necessities into a conceptualisation of time as a measure of social welfare. It is taken as given that everyone must spend a certain amount of time attending to the 'necessities of life': doing basic personal care tasks (sleeping, eating, bathing), performing minimal household tasks (cleaning, cooking, [for some] childcare) and working to live at or above the poverty line to afford food, shelter and clothing (Goodin et al., 2008: 34). This is largely beyond a person's control as the bare minimums are determined by biology (everyone needs to sleep), cultural norms (to do with cleanliness, for example) and the cost of living.

The amount of time left over after fulfilling one's basic needs and roles to a socially acceptable level is a person's discretionary time: the number of hours within a person's control for them to spend as they choose. Most people with 'temporal autonomy' or 'control over how one chooses to use one's own time' do not just spend this time resting (Goodin et al., 2008: 30). They also engage in hobbies or social activities. Long-term carer Millicent (60s, spouse with haematological cancer), for instance, spent an extra six to eight hours each week involved in community organisations.

Those people without temporal autonomy who cannot afford (the time) to maintain 'socially acceptable' levels in these three categories (personal care, household tasks, income) are said to be below the 'time poverty' threshold (Goodin et al., 2008: 5). This concept helps social researchers to recognise someone like Joe's experiences of strain as a result of time-poverty. As a result of the household and personal care tasks he had to perform for his wife, Joe was only sleeping three hours a night. Thus, in units of discretionary time, Joe would accurately be defined as time-poor (not, for instance, leisure-time rich).

In discretionary time, necessity is separated from choice, thus this measurement of time is superior to those that only measure how time is spent. As Goodin and colleagues (2008: 84) explain, 'time poverty, like money poverty ... [should] be defined not in terms of actual expenditures, but instead in terms of necessary expenditures'. A person who has little in their savings account after a year of extravagant cocktail parties and fine-dining bills should not be considered poor (Goodin et al., 2008). Nor should a person who has little spare-time after a week of working late hours because they choose (not need) to work late be considered time-poor (Goodin et al., 2008).

Hochschild (2000), however, points out that choice in the number of hours a person works is often limited by social factors as well as need. In *The Time Bind* she highlights the gendered and classed reasons many people work longer hours. For some it is a means of liberation from doing household chores. For others, working longer hours is part of a work culture that only takes executive employees seriously if they comply with working 40 or more hours each week. Szollos (2009) offers a further critique of the word 'choice' here. He argues that being time pressured is never an individual choice. Instead, 'time pressure is always an interaction between the person and the environment, and ... individual variations and context always need to be taken into account' (Szollos, 2009: 339).

Despite these limitations,[2] Goodin et al.'s (2008) overall conceptualisation is valuable and used here to understand variations in carers' emotional experiences. This argument that control over time matters more than time itself to a person's social welfare (Goodin et al., 2008; Szollos, 2009) guided my analysis of carers' experiences. Goodin and colleagues' conceptualisation of 'discretionary time'

---

2   Critiques related to 'choice' are arguably less relevant to an analysis of informal caregiving. The temporal demands of care work are less often determined by choice and more often determined by the patient's symptoms and mobility.

pushed me to examine, not just how much time each carer spent caring, but how much time they spent in their other roles and how much control they had over their time and commitments.

Time-Sovereignty

There was a significant difference in the experiences of those carers who could and those who could not choose to become more or less busy to either distract themselves from their emotions or attend to their emotions. This understanding of time and temporal autonomy informed my placement of carers' experiences into three categories: time-sovereign, time-poor and time-destitute carers (see Figure 5.1).

Time-sovereign carers were those carers, like Fred and Jane, who (x) were looking after a spouse whose cancer and treatment were not debilitating and (y) did not have other substantial 'claimants' on their time (Hassard, 1990: 12). Six males and seven female (41 per cent) fell into this category. For these carers, caregiving responsibilities were largely social and emotional, not physical, and took up only a moderate amount of their time. Because they did not have paid work or other caring responsibilities they had control over their time.

Time-poor carers were those carers, like Joe, who (x) were looking after a spouse whose cancer and treatment were debilitating and (y) did not have other demands on their time. Over 15 per cent (3 males and 2 females) fell into this category. These carers were providing many arduous personal care tasks such as bathing and lifting their spouses, in addition to giving social and emotional support. Often, this meant caregiving took place 24 hours, or close to it, each day. Like time-sovereign carers, these carers did not have paid work or other caring responsibilities, which allowed them to meet their spouses' numerous and often arduous care needs.

Time-destitute carers were those carers, like Anne and Sally, who (x) were looking after a spouse whose cancer and treatment were not debilitating and (y) had multiple claimants on their time. Three husbands and four wives (22 per cent) fell into this category. Their caregiving responsibilities for their spouses were largely social and emotional, not physical, and moderately time-consuming. However, the other demands on their time, including paid work, other caregiving responsibilities and childcare, left them with very little control over their time.

No interviewees fell into the category of (x) providing time-consuming physical care and emotional support to their spouse as well as (y) juggling multiple responsibilities outside of caregiving. Undoubtedly, if any carers' experiences match this description, they too would be qualitatively categorised as time-destitute.

These qualitative concepts exist on two continuums (see Figure 5.1). X represents the time-demands of caregiving, moving from left to right, from least to most demanding. Those providing social and emotional support are on the

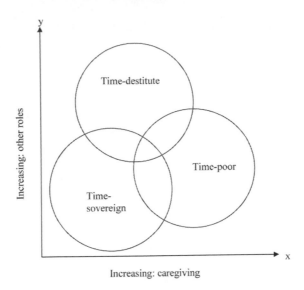

Figure 5.1   Categorisation of carers' autonomy based on (x) the time-demands of caregiving and (y) the time-demands of their other roles

left, categorised as providing mild to moderate support. Those carers managing biomedical aspects of their spouses' treatment (administering or monitoring reactions to medication), providing personal and physical care (bathing, toileting or lifting) to their spouse, in addition to giving social and emotional support, would be categorised on the right as giving moderately to extremely demanding care. Y represents the number of other claimants on a carer's time and the time-consuming nature of these claimants, moving from bottom to top, from one to many responsibilities. Those solely providing care to their spouse are at the bottom of the spectrum. Those involved in paid work and caregiving for their spouse would be in the middle. Those managing multiple responsibilities (childcare, caring for elderly relatives and paid work) would be at the top.

Seven carers' experiences fell in between categories. Bernard (50s, spouse with breast cancer), for example, was between time-poor and time-destitute, working full-time and providing physical and emotional care to his wife, with his son's assistance. Other carers' experiences changed over time. Charlie (50s, spouse with breast cancer), for instance, was time-sovereign during our first interview, but by our second interview his wife's condition had deteriorated: she was vomiting uncontrollably. Charlie was continuously cleaning up and thus, he became time-poor. Viewing carers' experiences on a temporal continuum allows for a scaled conceptualisation of carers' experiences as fluctuating with changes in the patient's wellbeing, mobility, reactions to treatment and changes in family, financial, and employment status.

Time to Feel

Categorising carers experiences based on time-sovereignty uncovered a qualitative difference in carers' emotional experiences and showed that time and emotions are intimately linked. Studies of dementia carers and cancer carers show that a benefit of caregiving experienced by some carers is growing closer to the care-recipient (Kramer, 1997; McNamara, 2001; Grbich et al., 2001; Thomas et al., 2002).[3] Analysing carers' experiences based on the amount of control they have over their time shows that this benefit is not experienced equally.

Time-sovereign carers, by definition had control over their time and thus, had time to feel. These carers had more time to experience a range of emotions related to caregiving and cancer. They had time to feel and reconnect with their spouse. Time-sovereign carers like Fred and Jane also had to work to manage their emotions. They alternated between attending to and distracting themselves from their emotions, the two basic strategies to dealing with emotions (Maex and De Valck, 2006). Some time-sovereign carers (such as Millicent) managed their emotions by managing their time: attending TAFE (Technical and Further Education) classes and church committee meetings to distract themselves from their emotions. Intermittent distraction from one's emotions was, it seems, desirable for these carers.[4]

Time-poor carers, who were managing one very demanding caregiving responsibility (caring for their spouse), also had enough time to share emotion-rich experiences with their spouses. Time-poor carers had little time to themselves. In order to keep on top of the housework, treatment management, appointments, coordination and caregiving, these carers often gave up personal time and sleep. Yet, time-poor carers reported having some time to feel. They reported having enough control over their time to prioritise sharing emotions with their spouse and feel a reconnection or heightened sense of closeness with their spouse as a result of the cancer experience.

Those carers who were time-destitute had little control over their time due to the number and time-intensity of the multiple roles they were juggling. Consequently, these carers had little time to feel, as Anne and Sally's stories illustrate. Managing all of these commitments made it difficult for these carers to prioritise their own emotions. They had little time to themselves to sort through their emotions and little time to grow closer to their spouse.

---

3   One carer qualified, however, that this benefit depends, for spouse cancer carers, on the quality of the relationship before diagnosis. 'It just polarises things that are already on the ground' (Leo, 60s, spouse with breast cancer). If there is tension in the marriage before cancer, it may prompt divorce. If there is love and stability, cancer caregiving may help the relationship to grow stronger.

4   Too much distraction, however, could be problematic as evidenced by the experiences of time-destitute carers presented here.

Time for Support

In addition to facilitating understanding of emotional differences in cancer carers' experiences, time-sovereignty also explained variation in interviewees' support preferences. All carers in this study sought informal support, with varying success. The temporal quality of their caregiving experience shaped their formal support preferences. Time-sovereign carers, on the whole, tended to access emotion-focused support, such as counselling and support groups, while time-poor or time-destitute carers tended to prioritise financial or respite support.

Informal Support

All carers in this study sought the support of friends and family. In addition to traditional practical support, including chores, respite and medical advice, many carers reported seeking out conversations with friends or family to distract themselves from their emotions or to help them overcome their emotional confusion.

Sometimes, family and friends who lived close by took on some chores and responsibilities such as ironing, childcare, yard work and farm work. Neighbours, church friends and family often cooked for the carer and patient. One friend even replaced the patient's bedside flowers regularly. Doing these tasks allowed the carer more time to care or perhaps some time to be alone.

Periodically spending time with the patient was another way local friends and family helped the carer. It allowed the carer some respite from ongoing emotion management and assured the carer that a backup existed if required. Bernard's (50s, spouse with breast cancer) adult son, for example, would stop by in the afternoons to check on his mother. This helped Bernard to feel less anxious about his wife's health while he was at work. Conversely, losing a source of respite could be detrimental to a carer's sense of wellbeing. Andrew's son moved to another part of the country, provoking a surge in Andrew's anxiety until his sister-in-law came to visit. Overall, family and friends who were able to provide auxiliary caregiving reduced carers' anxiety and the burden of care.[5]

Carers also sought contact with friends and family to provide a diversion from their experience of the emotional burden of caring. Visits during periods of high anxiety in particular provided welcome distractions and companionship. For instance, Millicent (60s, spouse with haematological cancer) said her daughters' company during her husband's final days helped the time to go by much faster. A dinner out with Andrew's sister-in-law helped him to temporarily forget his anxiety about his wife's surgery. Visits from friends and family provided welcome interruptions from loneliness and worried preoccupation.

---

5   This finding was also made by Braithwaite in her study of carers of older people with dementia. Being a carer with no one else to rely on for help in caregiving was statistically related to having 'poor mental health' (Braithwaite, 1990: 119).

Carers sought out friends and family with cancer or counselling experience for help in interpreting and shaping their emotions and in maintaining the energy necessary to provide ongoing emotional support. Patrick (50s), whose wife had breast cancer, spoke with friends whose wives had breast cancer to gauge what to expect from the disease and how best to manage his own and his wife's emotions. He talked to workmates whose wives also had cancer about 'where they are at', which allowed him to compare and project his wife's illness trajectory. He talked with other husbands at breast cancer related functions and learned how they were dealing with their new awareness of mortality, allowing him to measure the normalcy and appropriateness of his own approach.

Fiona sought out her daughter's help in quieting her frustration, understanding her husband's feelings and rallying the energy to provide him with ongoing positive support. Her husband Mark had prostate cancer surgery that resulted in ongoing incontinence for 18 months. The incontinence left him severely depressed. Fiona saw her main role as emotionally 'propping up' or 'bringing up' her husband. When he was so 'low' that it got her 'down', frustrated and ready to 'switch off' she would call her daughter, who has a counselling diploma. She said their other two children were 'supportive and very sympathetic' but she needed her daughter to 'pull [her] a bit further than that', to help her to see her husband's side and give her emotional support so that she could continue to manage her own and subsequently, her husband's emotions.

On the whole, support from friends and family reduced carers' task, time and caring burdens. Informal emotional support, both in person and over the phone or internet, provided carers with a welcome distraction. Several carers talked with experienced family and friends about how to approach the future and how to provide ongoing emotion work.

However, informal support was not an option for all carers, nor was it easy to access for others. For some carers, friends and family were too far away to offer meaningful support. For others, accessing informal support was challenging, with friends often feeling uncomfortable about offering support for fear of intruding.

Many carers reported practical and emotional informal support as essential to their ability to care. Others had either very little informal support available, or found accessing informal support onerous. Many carers who found informal support too difficult or insufficient at meeting their needs for emotional support sought the services of counsellors or support groups. The next section explores the experiences of those who sought out counselling.

Counselling

Forty per cent of interviewees accessed counselling (9 male, 5 female; 4 time-sovereign, 4 time-poor, 3 time-destitute, 2 in between time-poor and time-destitute), describing it as a much needed rest from emotion management. Counselling offered carers a place for honest communication about grief, stress and anger, which they often hid from their spouses. Linda (40s, spouse with bowel cancer) described counselling as 'an opportunity to have a bit of a cry for a couple of hours'. Counselling also helped her to understand her emotional response to the diagnosis and caregiving.

> They would say, 'So what is it you are most afraid of? What is making you angry?' Whatever it happens to be. Those questions allowed me to think out loud. Trained counsellors can do that for you, they can help give some sort of shape to the emotions you are dealing with, and I found that useful.

Many attended to find reassurance that their emotions and emotion work were 'normal' and appropriate: 'they were able to convince me that my reaction was perfectly normal' (Rodney, 30s, spouse with breast cancer). Anne (30s, spouse with glandular cancer) said her counsellor allowed her to 'have a bit of a rant and a rave and he just sort of gives me a coping technique and makes me see things a little differently'.

Others were warned that they needed to focus more on their own emotions. Bernard (50s, spouse with breast cancer), for instance, was told to take time out for himself to ease the intensity of his emotions. He was also given information on 'things you have got to watch out for' to keep from becoming depressed, clinically anxious or getting sick with a stress related illness.[6] Some were taught meditation techniques or prescribed medication to alleviate anxiety and depression. Overall, therapy provided carers with a break from emotion work and an emotion management consultation.

Those who did not access counselling often cited having sufficient informal support as their reason. Some cited not knowing counselling was available. Bernard (50s, spouse with breast cancer) did not discover that counselling was available until after he developed anxiety. Anne (30s, spouse with glandular cancer) only learned about a free counselling service for carers by chance from a co-worker, saying, 'Information is just not given out. I don't know who is supposed to do it'.

Support Groups

Nearly 44 per cent of interviewees attended a face-to-face support group, most often (7) a local cancer support group facilitated by a psychologist and open to patients with all types of cancer and their carers (6 male, 8 female; 8 time-sovereign, 3 time-poor, 3 time-destitute). Story-sharing and interacting was a primary focus of these groups. Others attended peer-facilitated diagnosis

---

6   A few carers were encouraged to change their orientation to the future. For example, Blake had started to drink more as a way of managing his depression. His psychologist said he was focusing too much on the future loss of his wife which was creating his 'vicious cycle' of depression. To help him continue to provide care, his therapist recommended he look positively on the time they still had together in the present instead of anticipating his wife's death.

specific (2 prostate cancer; 2 neurological cancer; 1 asbestos-related disease) support groups. These groups were described as information and networking oriented. Two carers attended a therapy-focused group support session organised by a hospital-based psychologist.

Reported benefits were similar to those of counselling. Support groups were described as a 'very safe' place for carers to express emotions without evoking pity, to learn about controlling emotions and more clearly understand their feelings. In support groups, carers found relief from ongoing emotion management. Judy (60s, spouse with asbestos-related cancer) said, 'I had a cry .... We did what women do and what men should do'. Jane (60s, spouse with prostate cancer) said, 'For two hours it was somebody else caring for him'. An important aspect of emotion-sharing in support groups was that it was devoid of pity: 'You don't feel as though you are whinging' (Cindy, 60s, spouse with prostate cancer). 'It wasn't what some people thought it would be ... morose and lets all get our violins out. We are all so sorry. It wasn't that at all' (Linda, 40s, spouse with bowel cancer). As Sharon explained:

> There is something about being able to talk with other people who have been there [and] done that, because you can talk about it [and it] doesn't sound like you are trying to go 'oh, poor me, give me some sympathy'. It's just sharing your life experience. You can't do that with healthy able-bodied people because they don't understand and they don't really know what's involved and it just looks like you are self-seeking.

Jane (50s, spouse with prostate cancer) made a similar assessment. 'There is no pity. It's just a really comforting environment with like people with like problems and you just talk about it quite openly ... I am not alone'.

Unlike counselling, support groups were social and an opportunity to laugh. Carers found in them a balance between joy and sorrow. They were also an opportunity to 'see how they've [other carers] handled it' (Judy, 60s, spouse with asbestos-related cancer) and 'pick up a few hints on what to do in certain circumstances' (Andrew, 60s, spouse with breast cancer). Carers learned emotion management through observation. Experienced carers saw support groups as opportunities to help new carers, to tell them about available support and share practical tips. Meetings also allowed carers to know that they were not alone and find 'companionship' (Linda, 40s, spouse with bowel cancer). In support groups 'you don't feel so lonely and you have got someone to talk to ... without feeling ... uncomfortable' (Frank, 70s, spouse with haematological cancer).

Learning practical information was another unique benefit of support groups. Carers learned about other support services and financial aid programmes and how to access them. Other carers explained how to do practical tasks more easily, such as cutting pills with a pill cutter. Many learned about the likely illness trajectory. Carers found support groups to be an empowering opportunity to compare notes on treatment, helping them to learn more about side effects and treatment alternatives that they might then discuss with their doctor.

Carers who did not attend support groups typically reported sufficient informal support, a lack of awareness, or a lack of time. Phyllis (50s, spouse with neurological cancer) described support as 'left to what *you* can find out'. Ian (50s, spouse with breast cancer) described the local support group as 'difficult to get to'. Matthew (30s, spouse with breast cancer) and his wife, for instance, could not attend a support group for breast cancer patients because she worked at night and looked after their toddler-aged daughter during the day. Other carers explained that support groups were not their preference. Some preferred a distraction from thoughts on cancer. 'I don't like sitting about sharing stories ... I find that depressing. I'd much rather go with the dragon-boat people' (Colleen, 60s, spouse with prostate cancer). Others preferred respite. 'Can someone look after her for 5 minutes? That is support to me. Not all that emotional ... rubbish' (Charlie, 50s, spouse with breast cancer). Male carers in particular said they were 'unreceptive' (Bernard, 50s, spouse with breast cancer) to support groups. Tyler (60s, spouse with haematological cancer) assessed support groups as too expressive, saying this would undermine his resolve to be strong for his wife. Kyle (40s, spouse with breast cancer) thought support groups involved 'pillows' and 'daisy-chains', whereas he was angry and wanted to 'scream and shout'.[7]

Practical Support

Carers with little control over their time preferred practical support in the form of respite or financial aid. Two time-poor carers, with arguably the most physically demanding and time-intensive care responsibilities, accessed respite care. Joe (60s, spouse with ovarian cancer) arranged to have a volunteer come two hours a week. Joe used the time to run errands and buy groceries. He shed a few tears when he talked about this service, reflecting on the generosity of both the volunteer and his wife.

> A respite carer ... came ... once or twice a week .... She was a lovely lady and she did much more than was asked of her. And one of the conditions of this was the respite person came in to sit with the patient to talk to them and keep them occupied so the carer could go off and do things. And but (crying) the lady that

---

7   This largely gendered stigmatisation of support groups (and counselling), supported by past research (Druhan-McGinn and White, 2004; Shaw, 1997), paints a lonely depiction of male carers' stoic masculinity. It seems most female carers feel comfortable seeking both informal and formal support to address their emotion management difficulties. Males, on the other hand, are less likely to access either informal or formal support. They are more likely to only have one confidant: their wife (Pruchno and Resch, 1989; Allen et al., 1999). When she can no longer perform the function when she becomes ill, the male carer is left with no one to talk with informally or formally.

came to us certainly, and it was made clear that that respite person wasn't to be expected to give a patient medications or to help them go to the toilet, things like that, but in [my wife's] case she ... had a bowel that wasn't all that regular after her initial treatment .... When something was due to be passed there was a great urgency about it. And there was one occasion when I was out and (crying) the respite carer had to do all that and clean up afterwards which is more than was asked – they swore each other to secrecy about it .... I only found out about it later on. My guess is because [my wife] realised ... so that ... I didn't have to be here constantly.

Phyllis (50s, spouse with neurological cancer) received six hours of weekly respite. As Phyllis's husband's neurological cancer altered his personality and mental capacity, Phyllis 'desperately needed' the respite. She felt trapped because she was not receiving intellectual stimulation from her relationship. She spent her six hours running errands, exercising and occasionally meeting with friends. Although she described herself as 'lucky', it was not enough.

I was lucky I got respite ... I got six hours off for the week which you feel really lucky to get, but when you think when it's 24/7 it's not a lot really. So ... at the end of it I ended up exhausted .... I had two weeks respite ... [when my husband went to] the dementia unit .... And you come back refreshed after two weeks break and think well I can care for him better because I have had a break, but you have to fight to be able to get that.

For time-poor and time-destitute couples especially, money and time were seen as two essential resources at odds with each other. Earning money took time away from caregiving; caregiving took time away from paid work and hence reduced their income at a time when it was more important than ever as a result of the loss of one earner and large medical bills.[8]

Although time-destitute carers were often in financial need, few accessed the aid available to them through Centrelink, the Australian welfare department. Only five carers accessed financial support available to carers (2 female, 3 male; 1 time-sovereign, 3 time-poor, 1 time-destitute). Many carers had not heard of the financial support available. Of those who knew of it, many were dissuaded by the onerous application process and insignificant amounts of money.[9]

Applying to Centrelink imposed its own time demands: many transactions had to occur in person and forms were long. The requirement that carers submit paperwork in person, 'no matter how sick' the patient was (Millicent, 60s, spouse

---

8   Supporting this qualitative finding, Braithwaite (1990) has also found that a lack of material resources is statistically linked with higher rates of psychiatric morbidity amongst informal carers of the elderly with dementia.

9   See Chapter 1.

with haematological cancer) was a deterrent. For Joe (60s, spouse with ovarian cancer), whose wife was in a wheelchair, this was no easy feat.

> After filling [the forms] out ... they wouldn't accept that they [paperwork for Centrelink] could just be posted in you had to take them in, in person .... I couldn't just leave her here and go down there so I had to get [my wife] out of bed, dress her, into the wheelchair, out to the car, into the car, put the wheelchair away, go down to Centrelink, get the wheelchair out, get [my wife] in, go there. And then stand in a queue at Centrelink.

Furthermore, the lengthy forms were described as 'appalling' (Marian, 50s, spouse with neurological cancer) and 'hard work' (Millicent, 60s, spouse with haematological cancer). 'Page after page after page you have got to fill out' (Marian). Linda (40s, spouse with bowel cancer) described this as conspiratorial.

> We are going to make it so hard for you to get this, at this probably worst time of your life. We are going to make you jump through all these hoops.

Kyle (40s, spouse with breast cancer) echoed her assessment.

> The thing I found really frustrating with Centrelink was the amount of repetition filling in forms, and I am sure they do it just to piss people off so they give up.

Carlie (50s, spouse with oral cancer) indicated the paperwork's exaggerated 15 cm thickness with her hands and said, 'I looked at the papers ... and I said no, no way! No, I couldn't be bothered'. After working all day and caring for her husband in the evenings, she had already had 'enough mental, emotional things now without fighting Centrelink'.[10] The application's length and degree of detail, including listing all gifts received, was a deterrent for many carers, especially those who were already time-poor or time-destitute. Many who needed the financial assistance or could have experienced less financial strain as a result of receiving it did not apply or put off filling out and submitting the Centrelink forms.

An additional deterrent for many carers was the 'confronting' nature of Centrelink questions, in person and on the application (Matthew, 30s, spouse with breast cancer). To receive financial aid, if the patient does not meet the physical limitation requirements, the carer and patient must emphasise that the patient has a terminal illness and hence a limited future. Following this path is 'negating that positive approach' that some carers, like Marian (50s, spouse with neurological cancer), followed. She followed complementary and alternative medicine recommendations of believing that they could slow the cancer's spread by doing

---

10   Similar sentiments have been expressed by carers in others studies (Dow et al., 2004: 27).

everything possible and truly believing that the patient would live.[11] 'Part of our mindset', she explained:

> Was: the only way we could beat this was by believing we could. So, getting a doctor to say we have only got three months was sort of negating that approach. So you can't have the both [optimism and Centrelink support].

Time-Sovereignty, Emotions and Support Preferences

This chapter offers another means of understanding differences in cancer carers' experiences, time-sovereignty, based on inductive qualitative research, underpinned by the sociology of time. Much of the literature in this field has been psychological and quantitative, with studies showing younger and female carers are more likely to experience caregiving as burdensome (Thomas et al., 2002; Thompson, 2005; Perz et al., 2011). The reasoning behind this variation is poorly understood. Time-sovereignty offers one potentially helpful schema for categorising carers' experiences and understanding their support preferences.

As demonstrated in Chapters 3 and 4, caregiving entails demanding emotion work that prompts many to seek guidance from friends, family, counsellors and support groups. Time-destitute carers, however, lacked time to explore their emotions. Understanding carers' experiences based in time-sovereignty uncovered a difference in carers' emotional experiences. A benefit of caregiving, growing closer to the care-recipient (Grbich et al., 2001; McNamara, 2001; Thomas et al., 2002; Ussher et al., 2011), is not experienced equally. Time-sovereign carers have time to reconnect with their spouse; time-destitute carers do not.

Further, this approach clarifies the correlations established in past research between age, gender and unmet needs. Findings support Burns et al.'s (2004) hypothesis that competing role claims may explain why younger carers have more unmet needs. Older, retired carers, with grown children tend to have more temporal autonomy (Goodin et al., 2008).[12] Older time-poor carers with an exceptionally taxing caring role are an important exception. Furthermore, women tend to have less discretionary time because they 'are responsible for juggling more roles inside and outside the family' (Northouse et al., 2000: 281).

---

11 See Chapter 3.

12 Having young children, especially under the age of five, has been found to increase the amount of time required to meet basic needs in all three of Goodin et al.'s (2008) categories: income, household chores and personal care. In Australia, this decreases a person's discretionary time by 13 hours, making young children the most significant contributor to a person's lack of spare time (Goodin et al., 2008). Furthermore, statistical analysis of the experiences of carers of older adults with dementia also supports this conclusion (Braithwaite, 1990: 80–87).

Their time is more centred on meeting the needs of 'significant others', restricting their time-sovereignty (Davies, 2001: 136).[13] Multiple demands on and lack of control over their time explains why younger female carers are statistically more likely to have unmet needs.[14] Thus, sociocultural, not just innate, characteristics illuminate much of the variation in cancer carers' experiences.

Findings also help us to understand cancer carers' support preferences. The reasons for variations in carers' support preferences are twofold: time-sovereign carers 1) have more emotion-rich caring experiences that more often necessitate accessing emotional support and 2) they can afford the time to access this emotional support. Previous research has been limited to carers generally, using psychological markers of efficacy (Boulton et al., 2001; Pearson, 2006). In this chapter I examine how support services are valued by carers of cancer patients in units defined by carers (Thomas et al., 2001; Herron, 2005). Counselling offered respite from emotion work. Support groups provided an opportunity to observe or share emotion management strategies and practical information, supporting Harding and Higginson's (2003) assessment of support groups. Time-sovereign carers with time to reflect on emotions and emotion-management often valued counselling and support groups. Respite and financial support were often valued by time-poor and time-destitute carers, but rarely accessed.

Thus, cancer carers' support preferences are largely dependent on time-sovereignty. Time-poor and time-destitute carers prefer practical support which gives them more time to juggle their competing roles or indeed, time to feel. Their primary focus was finding enough time to manage their competing responsibilities. Time-sovereign carers tend to prefer emotional support that helps them to organise, manage and validate their emotions and emotion work. Time-sovereign carers had so much time to feel that many made an effort to distract themselves from their emotions. They appreciated emotional support and distractions from friends and family via the phone and in other formats. They more often sought out help in managing their emotions.

Carers who did not access counselling or support groups gave four reasons: sufficient informal support, lack of time, lack of awareness or gendered perceptions of emotional support. Those who did not access practical support

---

13   The people to whom women attend to are not limited to children. Women are also more likely to be carers (ABS, 1999; Allen et al., 1999). Adding paid work reduces women's spare time considerably (Davies, 2001). Working mothers have approximately 30 per cent less spare time than stay-at-home mothers (Goodin et al., 2008). Conversely, male carers are more likely to have autonomy over their time because they are less likely to be looking after older relatives and children.

14   This conclusion is supported by results from both Fallowfield (1995) and Sherwood (2004). In their studies of cancer carers, they found that carers who balance more than one role, such as work and caregiving, more often experience caregiving as problematic. Statistical analysis of all carers' needs also shows a link between reporting higher rates of unmet needs and reporting 'negative effects on the [carer and care receiver] relationship' (Gibson et al., 1996).

described lack of time and lack of awareness as central reasons. Overall, the most time-poor carers seem to be the least able to access support because of the time and energy required to apply, long waits and bureaucratic hurdles. For some, another deterrent is the requirement that they replace their optimistic approaches to the future with prognostic pessimism in order to access financial support. The inaccessibility of financial support indicates that these time-impoverished cancer carers are under-supported and may be most vulnerable to the negative mental and physical health consequences linked to caregiving.

Conclusion

This chapter offers a qualitative and sociological approach, based in Goodin et al.'s (2008) concept of discretionary time, to understanding cancer carers' diverse needs, experiences and support preferences. Findings clarify an intuitive but poorly documented dimension of cancer carers' experiences and support needs: that time-sovereignty explains much of the variation in carers' emotional experiences and support preferences. Previous studies have been largely quantitative, focusing on age and gender in statistical analyses of unmet need. Time-sovereignty provides a new yardstick for understanding variation in cancer carers' emotional experiences and support preferences, offering health professionals a new means of tailoring support services and information to meet carers' needs. As these categories are fluid, however, this means carers' situations need to be continuously reassessed. Medical and psychosocial support personnel armed with this new way of conceptualising carers' experiences and needs can personalise offers of assistance.

Conclusion
Towards a Sociology of Cancer Caregiving

Caring for a spouse with cancer in the twenty-first century is an act and role plagued by uncertainty. No longer synonymous with death, cancer is now a reminder of life's limitations. It poses a 'cloud of metastatic possibilities' (Sally, 40s, spouse with bladder cancer) overshadowing a couple's taken-for-granted future orientation. This uncertainty makes contemporary cancer caregiving an especially important topic for sociological inquiry. Sociology, since its infancy, has focused on complexity and change: understanding the influence of industrial, technological, epidemiological and materialist shifts on individual narratives using a range of methods, theories and lenses. This book proposes a sociology of cancer caregiving and provides a micro-sociological analysis of cancer carers' experiences to begin the process of extending, complementing, and, in some instances, replacing the predominantly psychological and quantitative scopes of analysis that predominate in this field.

Cancer caregiving research to date has made the valuable contribution of a large number of quantitative studies into carers' needs. Carers and patients have differing needs depending on their stage in the cancer experience (Harding and Higginson, 2003). Upon initial diagnosis there is an urgent need for information and familiarity with medical systems before treatment. Following treatment, goals are geared more towards moving past the cancer experience. Recurrence and/or going into palliative care similarly invoke differing needs, with couples requiring less information and more emotional support (Harding and Higginson, 2003). Carers' needs also vary by age and gender.[1] Younger carers report less knowledge of available services, more burden, more emotional needs and greater unmet needs (Ciambrone and Allen, 2005; Sharpe et al., 2005; Burns et al., 2004). Older couples are more likely than younger couples to grow closer as carer and care-receiver (Thompson, 2005; Kramer, 1997). Female carers (particularly younger ones) report high levels of stress, burden, depression and unmet needs for respite care (Sharpe et al., 2005; Harding and Higginson, 2003).

Studies such as those reviewed in Molyneaux et al.'s (2011) convergent review of the literature have also established that few carers identify with the title. Most continue to identify as a spouse, friend, child or parent, despite their additional caregiving responsibilities. A lack of identification with the title, however, is associated with not accessing the social support available to carers (Hoffman, 2002). Research into support services for carers has established its effectiveness at reducing burden (Boulton et al., 2001).

---

1   See Chapters 4 and 5.

These studies, while significant in their contribution to the field, have been limited in their capacity to answer questions about why carers' needs vary by age and gender, why some embrace the title 'carer', what meanings spouses attach to their caregiving activities, how support services are beneficial to carers and why so few carers access them. Quantitative studies into cancer carers' needs are important, but limited because they use categories pre-determined by researchers in their analyses. Other studies, such as those into carers' identification with the label 'carer', are limited by their tendency to neglect diversity in carers' experiences (Greenwood et al., 2009) and their lack of theoretical engagement.

Sociology is well positioned to provide the methodological and theoretical tools required to make sense of the 'messiness' of caregiving journeys: the diversity in carers' experiences, roles and identities, the emotional ambiguity that accompanies prognostic uncertainty and the impact of uncertainty on a couple's cancer journey and orientation in time. As Remennick (1998: 7) explains, to 'unravel' the 'complex and multifactorial etiological webs' in which cancer patients and carers' experiences are wrapped, 'diverse research perspectives' and theoretical perspectives need to be applied. Qualitative methods, which hold a rich history in the sociology of health and illness, allow for participant-driven conceptualisations, using units defined by carers, and the prioritisation of variation. Qualitative approaches also facilitate exploration of 'why' questions, such as why some carers experience caregiving as burdensome and others as fulfilling. As Li et al. (2013: 185) explain in their review of the literature, 'there is no single best method to advance our understanding of couples confronting cancer', however, 'an in-depth understanding of the caregiver experience for cancer patients cannot be achieved from a quantitative study'.

Context is also central to sociological inquiry. The inclusion of the carer's whole 'story' in qualitative sociological research allows for in-depth insights and 'input from real-world situations' (Taylor and Dakof, 1988: 98). Thus, a sociological approach to examining cancer caregiving offers a wider scope of inquiry by analysing individuals and their social, cultural and temporal environments. Additionally, a sociology of cancer caregiving can offer a range of theoretical perspectives to the problem of understanding carers' varied, layered, gendered and contextual experiences. Sociological concepts of emotion, time and identity are particularly useful in this regard.

Towards a Sociology of Cancer Caregiving

This book aims to advance a sociology of cancer caregiving.[2] It illustrates the value of adopting an inductive and interactionist approach to examining carers' cancer journeys, showing the merits of applying sociological methods and

---

2   The use of the indefinite article 'a' rather than definite article 'the' is intentional. Rather than claiming terrain for a new speciality or subdiscipline within sociology (see

theories to reimaging cancer caregiving as varied phenomena shaped by social, emotional, temporal, political, historical, interactionist and economic forces – but actively responded to by carers. Based in inductive analysis of the stories of 32 carers of a spouse with cancer in one Australian city, I show that caring for a spouse with cancer often involves indefinite loss, a sense of confusion about complex emotions and contradictory emotion work, but little time to reflect on these emotions. I explore the complexities of carers' identities as both spouse and carer, and the impact of the process of prognostication on carers' and patients' shared orientations in time and subsequent emotion work. The findings foster new ways of conceptualising carers' experiences which will be of use to health and psychosocial support professionals seeking to tailor support for spouse cancer carers. The findings may also offer current carers of a spouse with cancer the sense of comfort that accompanies the reading of a shared narrative. In the paragraphs that follow, the contributions of this book to the sociology of cancer caregiving are summarised, followed by consideration of the potential drawbacks and merits of such an endeavour: normalisation and validation. The chapter concludes with macro-sociological directions for future sociologies of cancer caregiving.

Identities

Past research has regarded the term 'carer' as either a success or failure, imposing a bureaucratic lens. In the sociological analysis of cancer carers' stories presented in this book, a new appreciation of spouse carers' identities is offered using participant-driven methods and Holland et al.'s (1998) depiction of identities as fashioned by socio-cultural forces, but authored by individuals. Asking spouse carers for their stories, reflections on the term and perceptions of their roles permitted richer insights. Identification with the title 'carer', it was found, is relationally-situated and dependent on emotional interactions. Ironically, the title is meaningful in its lack of meaning. Carers' define it as a label for performing physical care tasks, often devoid of emotionally meaningful interaction with the care-recipient.

   With cancer, roles change. Spouses become patient advocates and managers of their spouse's care at home and in the hospital. Cancer carers also take on more of the household responsibilities: childcare, financial responsibilities and housework. Despite these changes, few identify as carers. Spouses often reject the title 'carer' as insufficiently encompassing of the emotional dynamics of their relationship to the patient and too bureaucratic. They prioritise their married identities as husband and wife, as long as there is sufficient emotional reciprocity in their relationship to maintain these spouse identities. If the capacity for meaningful exchange diminishes, if the patient can no longer 'give back' (Judy, 60s, spouse with asbestos-related

---

Mellor, 1992), the aim in this book is to demonstrate the need for and merits of taking a sociological approach to analysing carers' cancer journeys.

cancer) these spouses may identify as carers to position themselves as 'entitled' to support in interactions with medical and support professionals. Holland et al.'s (1998) concept of 'identity as practice' aids in recasting the debate about carers' identification with the title, making available a conception of cancer and marriage as two competing figured worlds. The encompassing nature of the figured world of marriage means that intermittent caregiving fits with ease within the parameters of this figured world; spouses need not redefine their roles, identities or relationships to accommodate for their new responsibilities and priorities. If the meaningful interactions and activities that comprise the figured world of marriage diminish, however, spouses are more apt to position themselves as carers within the figured world of cancer, authoring an identity as a co-worker and co-client. This inductive analysis of carers' stories and identification with the label 'carer' demonstrates the merits of furthering a sociology of cancer caregiving – a richer appreciation of the divergences in carers' experiences which offers professionals a potential indicator of increased burden and changed relationship dynamics.

Indefinite Loss

The psychological and death studies literature use the terms anticipatory grief and conventional grief, along with ambiguous loss, to communicate different forms of loss and grief occurring in the past, present and future. The inductive research presented here expands this literature. While anticipatory grief and conventional grief describe the experiences of a few carers, these terms do not match the loss described by most contemporary cancer carers in this study. Their loss had not yet occurred and it was not clear if and when it would. Thus, the term indefinite loss is offered to describe spouse cancer carers' uncertain and vacillating grief for a lost taken for granted future and consequently limited ability to plan for the future. Indefinite loss is a new concept afforded through a sociological and qualitative inquiry into cancer caregiving.

Coping and Emotion Work

Although loss is central to carers' experiences, it is not the whole of carers' emotional experiences. In contrast to the current cancer caregiving literature's focus on denial and coping, findings presented here suggest that carers of a spouse with cancer are typically not in denial and use different coping strategies at different times. Carers primarily coped in three ways: distraction, compartmentalising and escapism. Furthermore, interviewees' accounts show that cancer carers' use of coping strategies is typically only short term. To explore how cancer carers manage their own and their spouses' emotions in the long term, I employed sociologist Hochschild's concept emotion work. I found that carers manage patients' emotions to help them to be 'good patients', that is, to be positive and stoic. They did this through distraction, giving pep talks, listening, acting and blocking undesired communication.

Viewing emotions sociologically, as an ongoing and social process, uncovered the long-term patterns around temporal orientation in carers' and patients' emotion work. The diagnosis and consequent uncertainty about the future causes carers to experience what I refer to as *temporal anomie*. To overcome their lost sense of direction towards the future, carers either alter their temporal orientation or manage their emotions to maintain their current orientation. In line with advice from medical professionals, many carers manage their own and their spouses' emotions to be positive but realistic: to alter their focus from planning for a future together to enjoying life in the present. Others maintain a focus on the future by performing cognitive emotion work, either believing they would overcome the cancer or believing that nothing had changed, that their futures were never guaranteed. How medical professionals frame the diagnosis is central to the patient and carers' subsequent temporal orientation.

Using the concept temporal anomie and, following Thomas and colleagues (2001), Hochschild's (1983) concept emotion work to interpret carers' emotional experiences builds an interactionist platform for a sociology of cancer caregiving. The value of these concepts to understanding the emotional and temporal dynamics of carers' stories, and the influence of cultural expectations and medical interactions to their practices suggests the value of broad scopes of inquiry to the proposed sociology of cancer caregiving. Carers do not cope in isolation; emotions are interactive. Solely examining coping strategies is insufficient. Widening the scope to examine the influences of medical interactions and social support in understanding carers' emotions provides a more accurate picture of carers' emotions and doing so in future studies will help to decrease the misdiagnosis of denial and improve the quality of researchers' recommendations about how to support cancer carers. Furthermore, using interactionist theoretical lenses, such as 'emotion work' and 'identity as practice', permits the admission of both individual agency and structural forces in grasping carers' experiences, acknowledging the social determinants as well as the modicum of control these carers have over their journeys. Thus, rather than viewing carers as 'passive victims', these concepts foster appreciation of patients and carers as active creators of their cancer experiences, located within a sociocultural time and place (Thomas and Morris, 2002: 181).

Feelings and Conflicting Feeling Rules

In advancing a sociology of cancer caregiving, theoretical lenses can be useful in their capacity to help the researcher to see variations in data through different prisms. Hochschild's (1983) and Collins' (2004) theories of emotion, emerging from the interactionist tradition within sociology, offer clues into why carers' experiences are bifurcated. Conflicting roles and feeling rules provide one explanation for why some carers grow closer to their spouse following a cancer diagnosis while others experience burden, anxiety, stress and depression. A (negative) terminal prognosis fosters clear priorities: completing tasks associated with their spouse's care and sharing emotional energy-rich rituals with their spouse in the time they have left. These new priorities facilitate positive emotional energy experiences of pride and fulfilment, which, in the labour studies literature, has been found to prevent emotional exhaustion. Caring for a spouse with a terminal prognosis, where the symptoms of the disease impose depersonalisation on the relationship also fosters clear priorities, but the lack of emotional energy rich interactions robs the carer of the sense of pride or fulfilment that other carers of a spouse in the terminal stage experience, leading to an imbalance in emotional investments and returns, and emotional dissonance. An (positive) ambiguous prognosis fosters unclear priorities. The boundaries between their roles as carer and spouse are unclear. These carers are unsure of how long they will be carers because of the haziness of the disease's trajectory. Thus, they are uncertain about the longevity of their caregiving and in some instances uncertain about how they should feel. Unsure of when they can stop prioritising their caregiving role, carers of a spouse with an ambiguous prognosis experience guilt associated with conflicting roles and clashing feeling rules, which have been found to lead to burn out in the labour studies literature. Using the prisms of Hochschild's (1983) and Collins' (2004) sociological theories of emotion work and emotional energy offers a new possible explanation, beyond age and gender, for why some carers experience enhanced closeness while others find caregiving stressful and burdensome.

Time Sovereignty

Goodin et al.'s (2008) concept of discretionary time provides a sociology of cancer caregiving with another useful theoretical lens for understanding variation in carers' experiences. It fosters an appreciation of control over time as a measure of social welfare and another means of understanding differences in spouses' caregiving journeys and support preferences. Based in inductive insights and Goodin et al.'s (2008) theory, I categorise carers' experiences based on time-sovereignty and introduce the fluid categories of time-sovereign, time-poor and time-destitute as indicators of carers varying emotional experiences and thus varying needs. Those carers with few demands on their time as a consequence of their caregiving role being less onerous and as a consequence of having few other responsibilities outside of caregiving, are categorised as time-sovereign. Carers, whose spouse requires substantial help, as a result of impairment to their mobility for instance, are categorised as time-poor. Those carers who had many demands on their time as a consequence of juggling multiple roles, such as parenting, caregiving and breadwinning, are categorised as time-destitute. This categorisation allows an overall qualitative difference in carers' experiences to emerge. Those carers who are time-destitute have little time to process, absorb and reflect on their emotions. In short, unlike more time-sovereign carers, who tend to grow closer to their spouse, these carers have little time to feel, showing that free time is necessary to processing and reflecting on one's feelings.

Intersections in carers' emotions and time-sovereignty shape their support preferences. Time-sovereign carers, having more control over their time, have time to reflect on their emotions. Thus, these carers prefer emotion-focused support. Time-destitute carers, in contrast, have multiple claimants on their time, leaving them with little control over their time and little time to reflect and absorb their emotional responses to their spouse's diagnosis. Thus, they prefer practical (respite and financial) support, allowing them more time to complete their caregiving responsibilities and more control over their time. It is these services, however, that are the most stressful and time consuming to access. The onerous nature of applying for support is a deterrent to many time-poor and time-destitute carers. Thus, this book shows that the carers who could benefit most from accessing support services are in the worst position to access this support.

In sum, this book explores intersections across carers' lived experiences, laying the platform for a sociology of cancer caregiving. It offers a micro-sociological foundation, based in a range of interactionist theories, novel concepts and schemas. Holland and colleagues' (1998) theory of identity as practice allows for the reconceptualisation of cancer and marriage as two important figured worlds shaping carers' identity construction options. Hochschild's (1983) and Collins' (2004) interactionist sociological theories of emotions allows for insight into carers emotion management as dependent on emotional energy, priorities and roles as both family and carer. Goodin et al.'s (2008) theory of discretionary time as a measure of social welfare, fosters a richer understanding of the variations in carers' experiences and support preferences. New concepts, such as indefinite loss and 'positive but realistic' emotion work, acknowledge the social, cultural and temporal dimensions of carers' emotions. 'Time sovereignty' and identification with the title 'carer' offer new categories for understanding carers' varied needs and support preferences.

Normalisation and Validation

These innovative reconceptualisations, born from a sociological analysis of carers of cancer patients' narratives, have the potential to positively affect carers by guiding health professionals tailoring support for carers of cancer patients and offering carers a sense of validation. Concepts such as 'indefinite loss' arm support and psychosocial personnel with a clearer means of communicating the emotional experiences of carers of a spouse with cancer. They also bear witness to cancer carers' unique experiences of loss, providing validation and potentially helping carers to feel less alone.

However, some warn that these types of studies and findings can have a normalising and self-policing effect. Hutton (1988: 135), for example, argues that 'the self is an abstract construction, one continually being redesigned in an ongoing discourse gendered by the imperatives of the policing process' (as quoted by Frank, 1993: 49). He is arguing that individuals seek information on what is normal and either monitor themselves or are monitored by others to conform to this definition.

Others have argued that the social sciences are paramount in this process of conformity (Rose, 1989; Furedi, 2004; Powell, 2008). As Frank (1993: 49) explains, psychologists and sociologists provide 'types'. '"Types" then becomes "stages", and stage theories become institutionally enforced expectations'. Using the example of Elisabeth Kübler-Ross's (1969) well-known work with the dying, Frank shows how many social scientists seek to give 'voices' to different groups, but unintentionally propagate their regulation when the findings are 'appropriated in clinical settings to routinize how the ill are heard by staff, and even to label those who fail to conform to the "appropriate stages"' (Frank, 1993: 49). Thus, findings related to grief and emotions often become scales of normality for institutional and individual 'policing'.

Consequently, and for good reason, a person might conclude that sociological studies of cancer caregiving are problematic and pointless as they will only result in self or clinical regulation. I argue, however, that for several reasons that would be an example of the old German proverb, 'throwing out the baby with the bath water': discarding something valuable just because of a single (potential) fault.

First, findings such as the concepts presented here have the beneficial effect of 'giving a voice to the "other"' (Frank, 1993: 50), bearing '"witness" to the suffering' (Kleinman 1988; as cited by Bury, 2001: 282) and prompting action. Although Frank and Bury are referring to the suffering of patients, cancer carers' experiences may need witnessing even more so than patients, as they are often forgotten and in need of recognition by the media, by families and medical staff (Given et al., 2012; Given et al., 2006). In fact, this was one of the reasons many carers participated in the study. For example, in my field notes following my first interview with Anne (30s, spouse with glandular cancer), I wrote that she said 'thank you for doing this research. I just hope that it helps other carers to avoid what I went through'.

Anne's gratitude also speaks to a second value of these findings: legitimation (Bury, 1991). Compiling an overview of carers' loss, coping and emotion work gives credibility to their experiences. Reading accounts of other carers' emotional struggles can have the comforting effect of preparing others and decreasing their sense of stigma (Frank, 1993). Said in another way, people want to know that their experiences are shared by others (Gregory, 2005). A degree of self-policing is to some extent necessary because we are embedded social beings. Learning that others have gone through similar emotional experiences can be a relief and a source of validation. Learning about the range of emotions carers experience can help carers to stop asking 'what is wrong with me?' or 'why am I feeling this way?'

Describing the values of his illness narrative, Frank (1994: 16–17) says this yet another way.

My illness narrative tells a reader nothing more than what she has already experienced herself: why is it still of value? ... [because] The illness narrative addresses the desire to tell stories told many times before, precisely because they have already been experienced … . They should listen also for the desire to recognize and be recognized by others that these texts signify.

The terminology I offer in this book aids in this process of recognising and being recognised. Terms like 'indefinite loss', 'temporal anomie', and 'time-destitute' will be helpful to support service providers and carers looking for ways of identifying and communicating their emotional experiences.

Third, although studies on emotions run the risk of being fodder for regulatory and normalising efforts, recognising this risk may help to counter it. Warning social scientists and clinicians of the normalising potential that their practices hold may help to moderate their impact. For carers, acknowledging this normalising impact and the compulsion to conform may be empowering, by helping carers to recognise the constraints attached to their experiences (see Frank, 1993). Further, this research shows the variety of carers' experiences, as opposed to a description of *the* normal caregiving experiences. Highlighting the diversity in carers' experiences may also help to counter the tendency towards self-policing and policing within medical interactions.

Fourth, by using a sociological gaze, these findings highlight the external influences and constraints on carers' emotions, moving the implied action away from clinical regulation and self-monitoring. They have the potential to inform support services personnel of the structural constraints, such as time and money, on a carer's ability to process and reflect upon their emotions. They also have the potential to make both carers and medical professionals more aware of the interactionist nature of carers' long-term emotion work. It is a product of communication with the patient, doctors, nurses, counsellors and other carers.

In sum, although the findings and concepts presented in this book (as well as the conclusions of future sociology of cancer caregiving studies) risk having a normalising effect, they also have beneficial impacts, supporting an invitation to a sociology of cancer caregiving. 1) They 'give a voice' to cancer carers' often neglected experiences. 2) They help carers of a spouse with cancer to feel legitimated and prepared for the complex emotions and emotion work that lay ahead. 3) They inform professionals and carers of the normalising potential of this information. 4) They highlight the interactionist and external constraints on carers' emotions.

Future Directions

This book makes a substantial contribution to the advancement of a sociology of cancer caregiving. It demonstrates the novel insights to be gained from adopting an inductive and theory-rich approach to valuing carers' wide-ranging experiences. It suggests the value of these insights to carers – validation – and to support professionals seeking to shape support recommendations to individual carers, while acknowledging the danger of any study in which human experiences are categorised: self- and institutional policing.

This study is merely the second brick (Thomas and colleagues (2001) provided the first) of many needed to build a sociology of cancer caregiving and improve policy and practice for the under-recognised army of carers supporting their families (and medical systems) through cancer. Further research is needed, especially into the macro-sociological aspects of cancer caregiving. In closing, I offer a few suggestions for future sociology of cancer caregiving research: the cultural transferability of the concepts emerging from this book and carer wellbeing across political and organisational contexts.

Future research could explore the durability and applicability of the concepts presented here, such as time-sovereignty, indefinite loss and temporal anomie, across cultural, political and temporal contexts. Connell (2007) raises questions about the dominance of the (northern hemisphere) West in social theory and the transferability of sociological concepts across national, linguistic and cultural borders. Qi (2011), responding to Connell's questions, analyses the intersections and cultural departures in the Chinese concept of 'face' and Goffman's (1959) work on the presentation of self, demonstrating the importance of culture to sociological concepts. The sociology of time literature also suggests the economic relativity of orientations in time. Those in the middle-classes tend to take their future-orientation for granted, planning and saving for what seems like a secured future. Those with less material surety are likely to be present-oriented (Coser and Coser, 1990). Without assurance of where next week's food will come from, they are more likely to live for and in the present. The temporal impact of a cancer diagnosis may be more disruptive to those who are future-oriented – a contention that should be followed up in future research.

Further research should also explore the impact of differing organisational and political contexts on carer wellbeing. Several carers in this study depicted practical support services as limited, difficult to access and discouraging. Linda (40s, spouse with bowel cancer), for example, saw supporting carers as 'an important part of a caring community'. But, she described challenges in applying for financial support. First, 'knowledge about where to get financial support' is 'important', but difficult to find. Second, when applying for this support she said carers are made to 'feel as if you are trying to rort the system'. On the whole, she concluded that the agenda was to 'make it so hard to get this [financial support]. In this probably worst time of your life, we are going to make you jump through all of these hoops'.

The first challenge to accessing support is knowing it is available and how to access it. Linda was not alone in her assessment of information about support services for carers as sparse. In a recent survey conducted by Carers New South Wales (Broady, 2014), over a third of carers (36.3 per cent) described a lack of knowledge about available support services as a barrier to accessing support.[3]

---

3   This figure increases to 51.7 per cent for younger carers; over half of those carers surveyed who were under 35 years old identified not knowing about available services as a barrier to accessing support.

Future studies should explore carers' contact with different health and psychosocial professionals and organisations, to gain a richer understanding of how carers' (systematically or otherwise) learn about available support across different organisational contexts. Current pathways to support must first be established before these pathways can be improved in number and quality.

A second challenge to accessing support, particularly financial support, are the bureaucratic and political difficulties. Australian carers, such as Linda, are eligible for a Carers Payment and Carers Allowance, though accessing the support is often challenging and the financial support meagre. Carers are relied upon as 'resources' in Australia, but they are eligible for financial support as 'co-workers' and psychosocial support as 'co-clients' (Twigg and Atkin, 1994: 13).[4] This is not the case in all countries: some rely on carers more and provide less support (e.g. USA) while others provide sufficient institutional support to 'supersede' the need for carers (e.g. Sweden), though many patients still prefer to be cared for at home by a family carer. Future research should establish the impact of differing political contexts of care on caregiving experiences. Do Australian carers, on the whole, experience less burden than carers in countries without financial support and respite services available to carers? How much support is needed to affect burden and carer wellbeing? How do experiences of carer burden in Australia compare to experiences of burden in political contexts where carers' work is 'superseded' (Twigg and Atkin, 1994: 13) by the state (e.g. Sweden)?

Understanding the impact of organisational political contexts of care on carer wellbeing will be of paramount importance to policymakers as we weather the predicted swell in caregiving that will accompany our ageing population (Sinfield et al., 2012). Relying on family carers to treat patients outside of costly medical facilities is only more 'cost-effective' (National Cancer Control Initiative, 2003: 47) if carers are well enough to continue caring.

---

4 See the Introduction for an overview of differing political contexts of care.

References

ABS. (1999) *Disability, Ageing and Carers, Australia: Summary of Findings, 1998*. Canberra: The Australian Bureau of Statistics, Commonwealth of Australia.

———. (2011) *Life Expectancy Trends – Australia*. Canberra: The Australian Bureau of Statistics, Commonwealth of Australia.

———. (2013) *Disability, Ageing and Carers, Australia: Summary of Findings, 2012*. Canberra: The Australian Bureau of Statistics, Commonwealth of Australia.

Adam, B. (1992) Time and Health Implicated: A Conceptual Critique. In: Frankenberg, R. (ed.). *Time, Health and Medicine*. London: Sage.

Al-Gamal, E. and Long, T. (2010) Anticipatory Grief Among Parents Living with a Child with Cancer. *Journal of Advanced Nursing* 66: 1,980–90.

Allen, D. (2000) Negotiating the Role of Expert Carers on an Adult Hospital Ward. *Sociology of Health & Illness* 22: 149–71.

Allen, D., Griffiths, L. and Lyne, P. (2004) Understanding Complex Trajectories in Health and Social Care Provision. *Sociology of Health & Illness* 26: 1,008–30.

Allen, S., Goldscheider, F. and Ciambrone, D. (1999) Gender Roles, Marital Intimacy, and Nomination of Spouse as Primary Caregiver. *The Gerontologist* 39: 150–59.

Aubeeluck, A. and Buchanan, H. (2006) Capturing the Huntington's Disease Spousal Carer Experience: A Preliminary Investigation Using the 'Photovoice' Method. *Dementia* 5: 95–116.

Bard, M. (1997) The Price of Survival for Cancer Victims. In: Wiener, C.L. and Strauss, A.L. (eds). *Where Medicine Fails*. 5th ed. London: Transaction Publishers.

Baum, F. (2008) *The New Public Health*. South Melbourne: Oxford University Press.

Beaglehole, R. and Bonita, R. (2004) *Public Health at the Crossroads: Achievements and Prospects*. Cambridge: Cambridge University Press.

Beam, S.E. (2004) *Naked as We Came* [song]. Retrieved 17 December 2014 from: http://www.azlyrics.com/lyrics/ironwine/nakedaswecame.html.

Bella, L. (2010) In Sickness and in Health: Public and Private Responsibility for Health Care from Bismarck to Obama. In: Harris, R., Wathen, N. and Wyatt, S. (eds). *Configuring Health Consumers: Health Work and the Imperative of Personal Responsibility*. New York: Palgrave Macmillan, 13–29.

Benzein, E. and Saveman, B.I. (1998) Nurses' Perception of Hope in Patients with Cancer: A Palliative Care Perspective. *Cancer Nursing* 21: 10–16.

Blank, R.H. and Burau, V. (2014) *Comparative Health Policy*. New York: Palgrave Macmillan.

Blaxter, M. (2004) Life Narratives, Health and Identity. In: Kelleher, D. and Leavey, G. (eds). *Identity and Health*. London and New York, NY: Routledge.

Blum, K. and Sherman, D. (2010) Understanding the Experience of Caregivers: A Focus on Transitions. *Seminars in Oncology Nursing* 26: 243–58.

Boss P. (1999) *Ambiguous Loss: Learning to Live with Unresolved Grief*. Cambridge, MA: Harvard University Press.

Boudioni, M., Mossman, J., Boulton, M., et al. (2000) An Evaluation of a Cancer Counselling Service. *European Journal of Cancer Care* 9: 212–20.

Boulton, M., Boudioni, M., Mossman, J., et al. (2001) 'Dividing the Desolation': Clients Views on the Benefits of a Cancer Counselling Service. *Psycho-Oncology* 10: 124–36.

Braithwaite, V. (1990) *Bound to Care*. Sydney: Allen & Unwin.

Breitbart, W. (2006) Foreword: Communication as the Bridge to Hope and Healing in Cancer Care. In: Stiefel, F. (ed.). *Communication in Cancer Care*. Berlin: Springer.

Broady, T.R. (2014) *Carers NSW 2014: Carer Survey*. Sydney: Carers NSW, 70.

Broom, A. and Kirby, E. (2013) The End of Life and the Family: Hospice Patients' Views on Dying as Relational. *Sociology of Health & Illness* 35: 499–513.

Bruhn, J.G. and Rebach, H.M. (eds). (2014a) *The Sociology of Caregiving*. New York: Springer.

———. (2014b) The Contemporary Challenges of Caregiving. In: Bruhn, J.G. and Rebach, H.M. (eds). *The Sociology of Caregiving*. New York: Springer, 1–14.

———. (2014c) National Caregiving Policy Initiatives. In: Bruhn, J.G. and Rebach, H.M. (eds). *The Sociology of Caregiving*. New York: Springer, 185–99.

———. (2014d) Social Change and Caregiving. In: Bruhn, J.G. and Rebach, H.M. (eds). *The Sociology of Caregiving*. New York: Springer, 15–32.

Burns, C.M., Dixon, T., Smith, W.T., et al. (2004) Patients with Advanced Cancer and Family Caregivers' Knowledge of Health and Community Services: A Longitudinal Study. *Health and Social Care in the Community* 12: 488–503.

Burns, C.M., LeBlanc, T.W., Abernethy, A., et al. (2010) Young Caregivers in the End-of-Life Setting: A Population-Based Profile of an Emerging Group. *Journal of Palliative Medicine* 13: 1,225–35.

Bury, M. (1982) Chronic Illness As Biographical Disruption. *Sociology of Health & Illness* 4: 167–82.

———. (1991) The Sociology of Chronic Illness: A Review of Research and Prospects. *Sociology of Health & Illness* 13: 451–68.

———. (2001) Illness Narrative: Fact or Fiction? *Sociology of Health & Illness* 23: 263–85.

Capra F. (1982) *The Turning Point: Science, Society, and the Rising Culture*. London: Flamingo.

Carpenter, E.H. and Miller, B.H. (2005) Psychosocial Challenges and Rewards Experienced by Caregiving Men: A Review of the Literature and an Empirical

Case Example. In: Kramer, B.J. and Thompson, E.H.J. (eds). *Men as Caregivers*. Amherst, NY: Prometheus Books, 99–126.

Cash, B., Hodgkin, S, and Warburton, J. (2013) Till Death Do Us Part? A Critical Analysis of Obligation and Choice for Spousal Caregivers. *Journal of Gerontological Social Work* 56: 657–74.

Cassidy, T. (2013) Benefit Finding Through Caring: The Cancer Caregiver Experience. *Psychology & Health* 28: 250–66.

Chambers, M., Ryan, A. and Connor, S.L. (2001) Exploring the Emotional Support Needs and Coping Strategies of Family Carers. *Journal of Psychiatric and Mental Health Nursing* 8: 99–106.

Chiou, C.J., Chen, I.P. and Wang, H.H. (2005) The Health Status of Family Caregivers in Taiwan: An Analysis of Gender Differences. *International Journal of Geriatric Psychiatry* 20: 821–6.

Ciambrone, D. and Allen, S.M. (2005) Husbands Caring for Wives with Cancer. In: Kramer, B.J. and Thompson, E.H.J. (eds). *Men as Caregivers*. Amherst, NY: Prometheus Books, 294–313.

Collins, R. (1990) Stratification, Emotional Energy, and the Transient Emotions. In: Kemper, T.D. (ed) *Research Agendas in The Sociology of Emotions*. Albany, NY: State University of New York Press, 27–57.

———. (2004) *Interaction Ritual Chains*. Princeton: Princeton University Press.

Collins, R. and Makowsky, M. (1998) *The Discovery of Society*. Boston: McGraw-Hill.

Connell, R. (2007) *Southern Theory: A Global Dynamics of Knowledge in Social Science*. Crows Nest, NSW: Allen & Unwin.

Corden, A. and Hirst, M. (2011) Partner Care At the End-of-Life: Identity, Language and Characteristics. *Ageing & Society* 31: 217–42.

Coser, L. and Coser, R. (1990) Time Perspective and Social Structure. In: Hassard, J. (ed.). *The Sociology of Time*. London: Macmillan, 191–202.

Crouch, M. and McKenzie, H. (2000) Social Realities of Loss and Suffering Following Mastectomy. *Health* 4: 196–215.

Davies, K. (2001) Responsibility and Daily Life: Reflections Over Timespace. In: May, J. and Thrift, N. (eds). *Timespace: Geographies of Temporality*. London: Routledge, 133–48.

Davis, A. and George, J. (1993) *States of Health: Health and Illness in Australia*. Pymble, NSW: Harper Educational.

Davison, I. (2013) Govt Slammed Over Censored Caregiver Legislation. *The New Zealand Herald*. New Zealand: APN New Zealand Limited.

Department of Human Services. (2014) *Payment Rates for Carer Allowance*. Retrieved from: http://www.humanservices.gov.au/customer/enablers/centrelink/carer-allowance/payment-rates.

Docherty, A. (2004) Experience, Functions and Benefits of a Cancer Support Group. *Patient Education and Counseling* 55: 87–93.

Doka, K. (2006) Grief: The Constant Companion of Illness. *Anesthesiology Clinics of North America* 24: 205–12.

Dow, B., Haralambous, B., Giummarra, M., et al. (2004) *What Carers Value: Review of Carer Literature and Practice*. Melbourne: Department of Human Services and National Ageing Research Institute.

Druhan-McGinn, N. and White, K. (2004) *Toward best practice in supportive care service in the ACT*. Cancer Council ACT and ACT Department of Health and Community Care.

Duckett, S.J. (2004) *The Australian Health Care System*. South Melbourne: Oxford University Press.

Duckett, S.J and Willcox, S. (2011) *The Australian Health Care System*. South Melbourne: Oxford University Press.

Dufault, K. and Martocchio, B.C. (1985) Symposium On Compassionate Care and the Dying Experience. Hope: Its Spheres and Dimensions. *The Nursing Clinics of North America* 20: 379–91.

Duke, S. (1998) An Exploration of Anticipatory Grief: The Lived Experience of People During Their Spouses' Terminal Illness and in Bereavement. *Journal of Advanced Nursing* 28: 829–39.

Dumont, R.G. and Foss, D.C. (1972) *The American View of Death: Acceptance or Denial?* Cambridge, MA: Schenkman Publishing Company, Inc.

Elias, N. (1985) *The Loneliness of the Dying*. New York: Basil Blackwell.

Elison, J. and McGonigle, C. (2003) *Liberating Losses: When Death Brings Relief*. Cambridge, MA: Perseus Publishing.

Emslie, C., Browne, S., MacLeod, U., et al. (2009) 'Getting Through' Not 'Going Under': A Qualitative Study of Gender and Spousal Support After Diagnosis with Colorectal Cancer. *Social Science & Medicine* 68: 1,169–75.

Evandrou, M. (1996) Unpaid Work, Carers and Health. In: Blane, D., Brunner, E. and Wilkinson, R. (eds). *Health and Social Organization: Towards a Health Policy for the Twenty-First Century*. New York: Routledge, 204–31.

Fallowfield, L. (1995) Helping the Relatives of Patients with Cancer. *European Journal of Cancer* 31A: 1,731–2.

Fine, M.D. (2007) *A Caring Society? Care and the Dilemmas of Human Service in the 21st Century*. New York: Palgrave Macmillan.

Fine, M.D. and Glendinning, C. (2005) Dependence, Independence Or Inter-Dependence? Revisiting the Concepts of 'Care' and 'Dependency'. *Ageing and Society* 25: 601–21.

Fleischman, S. (1999) I Am ..., I Have ..., I Suffer from ... A Linguist Reflects On the Language of Illness and Disease. *Journal of Medical Humanities* 20: 1–31.

Folkman, S. and Lazarus, R.S. (1980) An Analysis of Coping in a Middle-Aged Community Sample. *Journal of Health and Social Behavior* 21: 219–39.

Frank, A.W. (1993) The Rhetoric of Self-Change: Illness Experience as Narrative. *Sociological Quarterly* 34: 39–52.

———. (1994) Reclaiming An Orphan Genre: The First-Person Narrative of Illness. *Literature and Medicine* 13: 1–21.

———. (1995) *The Wounded Storyteller: Body, Illness and Ethics*. Chicago: University of Chicago Press.

Frank, J.B. (2008) Evidence of Grief As a Major Barrier Faced by Alzheimer Caregivers: A Qualitative Analysis. *American Journal of Alzheimer's Disease and Other Dementias* 22: 516–27.

Frankenberg R. (1992) 'Your Time or Mine': Temporal Contradictions of Biomedical Practice. In: Frankenberg R (ed.). *Time, Health and Medicine*. London: Sage.

Freak-Poli, R., Bi, P. and Hiller, J.E. (2007) Trends in Cancer Mortality During the 20th Century in Australia. *Australian Health Review* 31: 557–64.

Frijda, N.H. (2000) The Psychologists' Point of View. In: Lewis, M. and Haviland-Jones, J.M. (eds). *Handbook of Emotions*. 2nd ed. New York: The Guilford Press, 59–74.

Fulton, G., Madden, C. and Minichiello, V. (1996) The Social Construction of Anticipatory Grief. *Social Science & Medicine* 43: 1,349–58.

Fulton, R. and Fulton, J. (1980) A Psychosocial Aspect of Terminal Care: Anticipatory Grief. In: Kalish, R.A. (ed.). *Caring Relationships: The Dying and the Bereaved*. Farmingdale, NY: Baywood Publishing Company, 87–96.

Fung, H.H. and Carstensen, L.L. (2006) Goals Change When Life's Fragility is Primed: Lessons Learned from Older Adults, the September 11 Attacks and SARS. *Social Cognition* 24: 248–78.

Funk, L.M., Allan, D.E. and Stajduhar, K.I. (2009) Palliative Family Caregivers' Accounts of Health Care Experiences: The Importance of 'Security'. *Palliative & Supportive Care* 7: 435–47.

Furedi, F. (2004) *Therapy Culture: Cultivating Vulnerability in an Uncertain Age*. Abingdon: Routledge.

Gallicchio, L., Siddiqi, N., Langenberg, P., et al. (2002) Gender Differences in Burden and Depression Among Informal Caregivers of Demented Elders in the Community. *International Journal of Geriatric Psychiatry* 17: 154–63.

Gauld, R. (2009) *The New Health Policy*. New York: Open University Press, McGraw Hill.

Gear, E. and Haney, C.A. (1990) The Cancer Patient After Diagnosis: Hospitalization and Treatment. In: Clark, E., Fritz, J.M., Rieker, P.P., et al. (eds). *Clinical Sociology Perspectives on Illness and Loss: The Linkage of Theory and Practice*. Philadelphia: The Charles Press Publishers, 274–88.

Gibson, D., Butkus, E., Jenkins, A., et al. (1996) *The Respite Care Needs of Australians*. Canberra: Australian Institute of Health and Welfare.

Gilhooly, M.L.M., Sweeting, H.N., Whittick, J.E., et al. (1994) Family Care of the Dementing Elderly. *International Review of Psychiatry* 6: 29–40.

Gilliland, G. and Fleming, S. (1998) A Comparison of Spousal Anticipatory Grief and Conventional Grief. *Death Studies* 22: 541–69.

Given, B., Given, C. and Sherwood, P. (2012) Family and Caregiver Needs Over the Course of the Cancer Trajectory. *Journal of Supportive Oncology* 10: 57–64.

Given, B., Sherwood, P. and Given, C. (2006) Family Support for the Older Cancer Patient. In: Muss, H.B., Hunter, C.P. and Johnson, K.A. (eds). *Treatment and Management of Cancer in the Elderly*. New York: Taylor and Francis, 587–610.

Glenn, E.N. (2010) *Forced to Care: Coercion and Caregiving in America.* Cambridge, MA: Harvard University Press.

Goffman E. (1959) *The Presentation of Self in Everyday Life.* New York: Anchor Books, Doubleday.

———. (1968) *Asylums: Essays on the Social Situation of Mental Patients and Other Inmates.* Camberwell, VIC: Penguin.

———. (1968) *Stigma: Notes on the Management of Spoiled Identity.* Ringwood, VIC: Penguin Books.

Goldie, P. (2002) Emotions, Feeling and Intentionality. *Phenomenology and the Cognitive Sciences* 1: 235–54.

Goodhead, A. and McDonald, J. (2007) *Informal caregivers literature review: A report prepared for the National Health Committee.* Wellington: Victoria University of Wellington.

Goodin, R.E., Rice, J.M., Parpo, A., et al. (2008) *Discretionary Time: A New Measure of Freedom.* Melbourne: Cambridge University Press.

Gould, S.J. (1995) The median isn't the message. *Adam's Navel and Other Essays.* London: Penguin Books.

Grbich, C. (1996) Theoretical Perspectives in Health Sociology. In: Grbich, C. (ed.). *Health in Australia: Sociological Concepts and Issues.* Sydney: Prentice Hall, 15–36.

Grbich, C., Parker, D. and Maddocks, I. (2001) The Emotions and Coping Strategies of Caregivers of Family Members with a Terminal Cancer. *Journal of Palliative Care* 17: 30–36.

Greenwood, N., Mackenzie, A., Cloud, G.C., et al. (2009) Informal Primary Carers of Stroke Survivors Living At Home – Challenges, Satisfactions and Coping: A Systematic Review of Qualitative Studies. *Disability & Rehabilitation* 31: 337–51.

Gregory, S. (2005) Living with Chronic Illness in the Family Setting. *Sociology of Health & Illness* 27: 372–92.

Guillemin, J. (1997) Planning to Die. In: Wiener, C.L. and Strauss, A.L. (eds). *Where Medicine Fails.* 5th ed. London: Transaction Publishers.

Guldin, M-B., Vedsted, P., Zachariae, R., et al. (2012) Complicated Grief and Need for Professional Support in Family Caregviers of Cancer Patients in Palliative Care: a Longitudinal Cohort Study. *Support Care Cancer* 20: 1,679–85.

Halvorson-Boyd, G. and Hunter, L.K. (1995) *Dancing in Limbo: Making Sense of Life after Cancer.* San Francisco: Jossey-Bass Inc.

Hamilton, C. (2010) *Requiem for a Species: Why We Resist the Truth About Climate Change.* Crows Nest, NSW: Allen & Unwin.

Harden, J. (2005) Parenting a Young Person with Mental Health Problems: Temporal Disruption and Reconstruction. *Sociology of Health & Illness* 27: 351–71.

Harding, R. and Higginson, I. (2003) What is the Best Way to Help Caregivers in Cancer and Palliative Care? A Systematic Literature Review of Interventions and Their Effectiveness. *Palliative Medicine* 17: 63–74.

Hardt, M. (1999) Affective Labour. *Boundary 2* 26: 89–100.

Harrison, J.P., MD. (1844) *Medical Ethics: A Lecture delivered 23 December 1843 before the Ohio Medical Lyceum.* Cincinnati: Enquirer and Message Print.

Hassard J. (1990) Introduction: The Sociological Study of Time. In: Hassard, J. (ed.). *The Sociology of Time.* London: Macmillan, 1–20.

Hemmings, C. (2005) Invoking Affect. *Cultural Studies* 19: 548–67.

Herron, L-M. (2005) Building Effective Cancer Support Groups: Report to the Department of Health and Ageing. The Cancer Council Australia.

Herth, K. (1993) Hope in the Family Caregiver of Terminally Ill People. *Journal of Advanced Nursing* 18: 538–48.

Hochschild, A.R. (1979) Emotion Work, Feeling Rules, and Social Structure. *The American Journal of Sociology* 85: 551–75.

———. (1983) *The Managed Heart.* Berkeley, CA: University of California Press.

———. (2000) *The Time Bind: When Work Becomes Home and Home Becomes Work.* New York: Henry Holt and Company.

———. (2012) *The Outsourced Self: Intimate Life in Market Times.* New York: Metropolitan Books: Henry Holt and Company.

Hodges, L.J., Humphries, G. and Macfarlane, G. (2005) A Meta-Analytic Investigation of the Relationship Between the Psychological Distress of Cancer Patients and Their Carers. *Social Science & Medicine* 60: 1–12.

Hoffman, M.K. (2002) Self-Awareness in Family Caregiving. *The Family Caregiver Self-Awareness and Empowerment Project.* Kensington, MD: National Family Caregiver Association and National Alliance for Caregiving.

Holland, D., Lachicotte, W., Skinner, D., et al. (1998) *Identity and Agency in Cultural Worlds.* Cambridge, MA: Harvard University Press.

Hughes, J. (2007) Caring for Carers: The Financial Strain of Caring. *Family Matters* 76: 32–3.

Hunt, M. (1991) The Identification and Provision of Care for the Terminally Ill at Home by 'Family' Members. *Sociology of Health & Illness* 13: 375–95.

Huynh, M., Alderson, M. and Thomson, M. (2008) Emotional Labour Underlying Caring: An Evolutionary Concept Analysis. *Journal of Advanced Nursing* 64: 195–208.

Irvine, R. (1996) Losing Patients: Health Care Consumers, Power and Sociocultural Change. In: Grbich, C. (ed.). *Health in Australia: Sociological Concepts and Issues.* Sydney: Prentice Hall, 191–214.

Jalland, P. (2006) *Changing Ways of Death in Twentieth Century Australia: War, Medicine and the Funeral Business.* Sydney: University of New South Wales Press.

Jansma, F.F.I., Schure, L.M. and Meyboom de Jong, B. (2005) Support Requirements for Caregivers of Patients with Palliative Cancer. *Patient Education and Counseling* 58: 182–6.

Johansson, L., Long, H. and Parker, M.G. (2011) Informal Caregiving for Elders in Sweden: An Analysis of Current Policy Developments. *Journal of Aging & Social Policy* 23: 335–53.

Jutel, A.G. and Dew, K. (2014) Introduction. In: Jutel, A.G. and Dew, K. (eds). *Social Issues in Diagnosis: An Introduction for Students and Clinicians.* Baltimore: Johns Hopkins University Press, 1–14.

Kalich, D. and Brabant, S. (2006) A Continued Look At Doka's Grieving Rules: Deviance and Anomie as Clinical Tools. *Omega: Journal of Death and Dying* 53: 227–41.

Kearney, N., Hubbard, G., Forbat, L., et al. (2007) *Developing cancer services: Patient and carer experiences.* Stirling: Cancer Care Research Centre, University of Stirling.

Kellehear, A. (1984) Are We a Death-Denying Society? A Sociological Review. *Social Science & Medicine* 18: 713–23.

———. (2007) *A Social History of Dying.* Cambridge: Cambridge University Press.

Kelly, B., Edwards, P., Synott, R., et al. (1999) Predictors of Bereavement Outcome for Family Carers of Cancer Patients. *Psycho-Oncology* 8: 237–49.

Kelly, K. and Christou, E. (2009) Policy, Politics and Family Caregiving. *Aging Today* 30: 7–9.

Kennedy, V. and Lloyd-Williams, M. (2006) Maintaining Hope: Communication in Palliative Care. In: Stiefel, F. (ed.). *Communication in Cancer Care.* Berlin: Springer.

Khan, N.F., Harrison, S., Rose, P.W., et al. (2012) Interpretation and Acceptance of the Term 'Cancer Survivor': A United Kingdom-Based Qualitative Study. *European Journal of Cancer Care* 21: 177–86.

King, D. (2012) It's Frustrating! Managing Emotional Dissonance in Aged Care Work. *Australian Journal of Social Issues* 47: 51–70.

Kleinman, A. (2012) The Art of Medicine. *Lancet* 380: 1,550–51.

Kramer, B.J. (1997) Differential Predictors of Strain and Gain Among Husbands Caring for Wives with Dementia. *The Gerontologist* 37: 239–49.

———. (1997) Gain in the Caregiving Experience: Where Are We? What Next? *The Gerontologist* 37: 218–32.

Kübler-Ross, E. (1969) *On Death and Dying.* New York: Macmillan Publishing Company.

Kutner, G. (2001) *Caregiver identification study.* Washington, DC: American Association of Retired Persons.

Laizner, A.M., Yost, L.M.S., Barg, F.K., et al. (1993) Needs of Family Caregivers of Persons with Cancer: A Review. *Seminars in Oncology Nursing* 9: 114–20.

Lee, R. and Ashforth, B. (1996) A Meta-Analytic Examination of the Correlates of the Three Dimensions of Job Burn-Out. *Journal of Applied Psychology* 81: 123–33.

Lewis, J.D. and Weigart, A.J. (1990) The Structures and Meanings of Social-Time. In: Hassard, J. (ed.). *The Sociology of Time.* London: Macmillan, 77–101.

Lewis, S. (2006) Caregiving. *Women's Health Seminar Series.* Bethesda, MD.

Li, Q.P., Mak, Y.W. and Loke, A.Y. (2013) Spouses' Experience of Caregiving for Cancer Patients: A Literature Review. *International Nursing Review* 60: 178–87.

Lin, I-F., Fee, H.R. and Wu, H-S. (2012) Negative and Positive Caregiving Experiences: a Closer Look At the Intersection of Gender and Relationship. *Family Relations: Interdisciplinary Journal of Applied Family Studies* 61: 343–58.

Lindemann, E. (1944) Symptomatology and Management of Acute Grief. *American Journal of Psychiatry* 101: 141–8.

Little, M. (1995) *Humane Medicine*. Cambridge: Cambridge University Press.

Little, M., Jordens, C., Paul, K., et al. (1998) Liminality: A Major Category of the Experience of Cancer Illness. *Social Science & Medicine* 47: 1,485–94.

Little, M., Jordens, C., Paul, K., et al. (2001) *Surviving Survival: Life After Cancer*. Marrickville, NSW: Choice Books.

Lois, J. (2006) Role Strain, Emotion Management, and Burnout: Homeschooling Mothers' Adjustment to the Teacher Role. *Symbolic Interaction* 29: 507–30.

Maex, E. and De Valck, C. (2006) Key Elements of Communication in Cancer Care. In: Stiefel, F. (ed.). *Communication in Cancer Care*. Berlin: Springer.

Mamo, L. (1999) Death and Dying: Confluences of Emotion and Awareness. *Sociology of Health & Illness* 21: 13–36.

Marwit, S.J., Chibnall, J.T., Sougherty, R., et al. (2008) Assessing Pre-Death Grief in Cancer Caregivers Using the Marwit-Meuser Caregiver Grief Inventory (MM-CGI). *Psycho-Oncology* 17: 300–303.

Massumi, B. (2002) *Parables for the Virtual: Movement, Affect, Sensation*. London: Duke University Press.

McKeown, T. (1979) *The Role of Medicine: Dream, Mirage or Nemesis?* Oxford: Blackwell.

McNamara, B. (2000) Dying of Cancer. In: Kellehear, A. (ed.). *Death and Dying in Australia*. South Melbourne: Oxford University Press, 133–44.

———. (2001) *Fragile Lives: Death, Dying and Care*. Buckingham: Open University Press.

McNamara, B. and Rosenwax, L. (2007) The Mismanagement of Dying. *Health Sociology Review* 16: 373–83.

Mead, G.H. (2000) Mind, self and society. In: Farganis, J. (ed.). *Readings in Social Theory: The Classic Tradition to Post-Modernism*. Boston: McGraw-Hill, 160–78.

Mellor, P.A. (1992) Death in High Modernity: The Contemporary Presence and Absence of Death. *The Sociological Review* 40: 11–30.

Meuser, T.M. and Marwit, S.J. (2001) A Comprehensive, Stage-Sensitive Model of Grief in Dementia Caregiving. *The Gerontologist* 41: 658–70.

Miller, J.F. (2007) Hope: A Construct Central to Nursing. *Nursing Forum* 42: 12–19.

Molyneaux, V., Butchard, S., Simpson, J., et al. (2011) Reconsidering the Term 'Carer': A Critique of the Universal Adoption of the Term 'Carer'. *Ageing and Society* 31: 422–37.

Montgomery, R.J.V. and Kosloski, K.D. (2014) Pathways to a Caregiver Identity and Implications for Support Services. In: Bruhn, J.G. and Rebach, H.M. (eds). *The Sociology of Caregiving*. New York: Springer, 131–56.

Morris, S. and Thomas, C. (2002) The Need to Know: Informal Carers and Information. *European Journal of Cancer Care* 11: 183–7.

Mutch, K. (2010) In Sickness and in Health: Experience of Caring for a Spouse with MS. *British Journal of Nursing* 19: 214–19.

Mystakidou, K., Tsilika, E., Parpa, E., et al. (2006) Demographic and Clinical Predictors of Preparatory Grief in a Sample of Advanced Cancer Patients. *Psycho-Oncology* 15: 828–33.

Nash, M.L. (1980) Dignity of Person in the Final Phase of Life: An Exploratory Study. In: Kalish, R.A. (ed.). *Caring Relationships: The Dying and the Bereaved*. Farmingdale, NY: Baywood Publishing Company, 62–70.

Nathan, L.E. (1990) Coping with Uncertainty: Family Members Adaptions During Cancer Remission. In: Clark, E., Fritz, J.M., Rieker, P.P., et al. (eds). *Clinical Sociology Perspectives on Illness and Loss: The Linkage of Theory and Practice*. Philadelphia: The Charles Press Publishers, 109–15.

National Cancer Control Initiative. (2003) *Optimising cancer care in Australia*. Clinical Oncological Society of Australia, The Cancer Council Australia and National Cancer Control Initiative.

Neimeyer, R.A., Prigerson, H.G. and Davies, B. (2002) Mourning and Meaning. *American Behavioral Scientist* 46: 235–51.

Netto, G. (1998) 'I forget myself': The Case for the Provision of Culturally Sensitive Respite Services for Minority Ethnic Carers of Older People. *Journal of Public Health Medicine* 20: 221–6.

New Zealand Ministry of Health. (2014) *Funded Family Care Notice and Operational Policy*. Retrieved from: http://www.health.govt.nz/our-work/disability-services/disability-projects-and-programmes/funded-family-care-notice-and-operational-policy.

Northouse, L.L., Mood, D., Templin, T., et al. (2000) Couples' Patterns of Adjustment to Colon Cancer. *Social Science & Medicine* 50: 271–84.

Oakley, A. (1985) *Sex, Gender and Society*. Aldershot: Gower.

Olson, R.E. (2011) Managing Hope, Denial or Temporal Anomie? Informal Cancer Carers' Accounts of Spouses' Cancer Diagnoses. *Social Science & Medicine* 73: 904–11.

———. (2012) Is Cancer Care Dependant On Informal Carers? *Australian Health Review* 36: 254–7.

———. (2014a) Exploring Identity in the 'Figured Worlds' of Cancer Care-Giving and Marriage in Australia. *Health and Social Care in the Community*.

————. (2014b) A Time-Sovereignty Approach to Understanding Carers of Cancer Patients' Experiences and Support Preferences. *European Journal of Cancer Care* 23: 239–48.

————. (2014c) Indefinite Loss: the Experiences of Carers of a Spouse with Cancer. *European Journal of Cancer Care* 23: 553–61.

Olson, R.E. and Connor, J. (2014) When They Don't Die: Prognosis Ambiguity, Role Conflict and Emotion Work in Cancer Care. *Journal of Sociology*.

Opie, A. (1992) *There's Nobody There: Community Care of Confused Older People*. Auckland: Oxford University Press.

Owen, D.C. (1989) Nurses' Perspectives On the Meaning of Hope in Patients with Cancer: A Qualitative Study. *Oncology Nursing Forum* 16: 75–9.

Pearson, A. (2006) *A Strategic Development Plan to Improve Supportive Care for People Living with Cancer*. Adelaide: Joanna Briggs Institute.

Perz, J., Ussher, J., Butow, P., et al. (2011) Gender Differences in Cancer Carer Psychological Distress: An Analysis of Moderators and Mediators. *European Journal of Cancer Care* 20: 610–19.

Petersen, A.R. (1994) *In a Critical Condition: Health and Power Relations in Australia*. St. Leonards, NSW: Allen & Unwin.

Pezzullo, L., McKibbin, R., Cheung, S., et al. (2010) *The economic value of informal care in 2010*. Canberra: Access Economics & Carers Australia.

Pine, V.R. (1980) Social Organization and Death. In: Kalish, R.A. (ed.). *Death, Dying, Transcending*. Farmingdale, NY: Baywood Publishing Company, Inc., 88–92.

Powell, J.L. (2008) Social Theory and Emotion: Sociological Excursions. *International Journal of Sociology and Social Policy* 28: 394–407.

Poynton, C. and Lee, A. (2011) Affect-Ing Discourse: Towards An Embodied Discourse Analytics. *Social Semiotics* 21: 633–44.

Prosser, B. and Olson, R. (2013) Changes in Professional Human Care Work: the Case of Nurse Practitioners in Australia. *Health Sociology Review* 22: 422–32.

Pruchno, R. and Resch, N. (1989) Husbands and Wives As Caregivers: Antecedents of Depression and Burden. *The Gerontologist* 29: 159–65.

Qi, X. (2011) Face: A Chinese Concept in a Global Sociology. *Journal of Sociology* 47: 279–95.

Radley, A. (1999) The Aesthetics of Illness: Narrative, Horror and the Sublime. *Sociology of Health & Illness* 21: 778–96.

Rando, T. (1988) Anticipatory Grief: the Term is a Misnomer But the Phenomenon Exists. *Journal of Palliative Care* 4: 70–73.

————. (2000) *Clinical Dimensions of Anticipatory Mourning*. Champaign, IL: Research Press.

Remennick, L. (1998) Introduction: the Cancer Problem in Medical Sociology and Demography. *Current Sociology* 46: 1–9.

Roberts, K. (2002) Are Long or Unsocial Hours of Work Bad for Leisure? In: Crow, G. and Heath, S. (eds). *Social Conceptions of Time: Structure and Process in Work and Everyday Life*. New York: Palgrave Macmillan, 165–78.

Rose, K.E., Webb, C. and Waters, K. (1997) Coping Strategies Employed by Informal Carers of Terminally Ill Cancer Patients. *Journal of Cancer Nursing* 1: 126–33.

Rose, N. (1989) *Governing the Soul: The Shaping of the Private Self.* London: Routledge.

Roth, J.A. (1963) *Timetables: Structuring the Passage of Time in Hospital Treatment and Other Careers.* New York: Bobbs-Merrill Company, Inc.

Saad, K., Hartman, J., Ballard, C., et al. (1995) Coping by the Carers of Dementia Sufferers. *Age and Ageing* 24: 495–8.

Sabo, D. (1990) Men, Death Anxiety, and Denial: Critical Feminist Interpretations of Adjustment to Mastectomy. In: Clark, E., Fritz, J.M., Rieker, P.P., et al. (eds). *Clinical Sociology Perspectives on Illness and Loss: The Linkage of Theory and Practice.* Philadelphia: The Charles Press Publishers, 71–84.

Salander, P. and Moynihan, C. (2010) Facilitating Patients' Hope Work Through Relationship: A Critique of the Discourse of Autonomy. In: Harris, R., Wathen, N. and Wyatt, S. (eds). *Configuring Health Consumers: Health Work and the Imperative of Personal Responsibility.* New York: Palgrave Macmillan, 113–25.

Sanders, S., Ott, C.H., Kelber, S.T., et al. (2008) The Experience of High Levels of Grief in Caregivers of Persons with Alzheimer's Disease and Related Dementia. *Death Studies* 32: 495–523.

Schwalbe, M. (2007) Emile Durkheim and Erving Goffman Meet Dr. Magneto. *Contemporary Sociology* 36: 210–14.

Shakespeare, W. ([1597] 1993) *Romeo and Juliet.* Mineola, NY: Dover Publications.

Sharpe, L., Butow, P., Smith, C., et al. (2005) The Relationship Between Available Support, Unmet Needs and Caregiver Burden in Patients with Advanced Cancer and Their Carers. *Psycho-Oncology* 14: 102–14.

Shaw, J. (1997) *Even if I Videoed This, No-One Would Believe Me.* Bendigo: Bendigo Health Care Group and Department of Health Services.

Sherwood, P.R., Given, B.A., Doorenbos, A.Z., et al. (2004) Forgotten Voices: Lessons from Bereaved Caregivers of Persons with a Brain Tumour. *International Journal of Palliative Nursing* 10: 76–83.

Short, S.D., Sharman, E. and Speedy, S. (1993) *Sociology for Nurses: An Australian Introduction.* Crows Nest, NSW: Macmillan Education Australia.

Sinfield, P., Baker, R., Ali, S., et al. (2012) The Needs of Carers of Men with Prostate Cancer and Barriers and Enablers to Meeting Them: A Qualitative Study in England. *European Journal of Cancer Care* 21: 527–34.

Sjolander, C. and Ahlstrom, G. (2012) The Meaning and Validation of Social Support Networks for Close Family of Persons with Advanced Cancer. *BMC Nursing* 11: 17–30.

Skene, L. (1990) *You, Your Doctor and the Law.* Melbourne: Oxford University Press.

Small, W. (1996) Emotion Work. In: Grbich, C. (ed.). *Health in Australia: Sociological Concepts and Issues.* Sydney: Prentice Hall, 263–87.

Smith, R. (2014) Dying of Cancer is the Best Death. *BMJ Blogs*, 31 December 2014. Retrieved 2 January 2015 from: http://blogs.bmj.com/bmj/2014/2012/2031/richard-smith-dying-of-cancer-is-the-best-death/.

Sontag, S. (1991) *Illness as Metaphor and AIDS and its Metaphors*. London: Penguin Books.

Soothill, K., Morris, S., Harman, J., et al. (2001) Informal Carers of Cancer Patients: What Are Their Unmet Psychosocial Needs? *Health & Social Care in the Community* 9: 464–75.

Sörensen, S., Pinquart, M. and Duberstein, P. (2002) How Effective Are Interventions with Caregivers? An Updated Meta-Analysis. *The Gerontologist* 42: 356–72.

Sourkes, B.M. (1982) *The Deepening Shade: Psychological Aspects of Life-Threatening Illness*. Pittsburgh: University of Pittsburgh Press.

Stacey, J. (1997) *Teratologies: A Cultural Study of Cancer*. London: Routledge.

Stetz, K.M. and Brown, M-A. (2004) Physical and Psychosocial Health in Family Caregiving: A Comparison of AIDS and Cancer Caregivers. *Public Health Nursing* 21: 533–40.

Stiefel, F. and Razavi, D. (2006) Informing About Diagnosis, Relapse and Progression of Disease – Communication with the Terminally Ill Cancer Patient. In: Stiefel, F. (ed.). *Communication in Cancer Care*. Berlin: Springer, pp. 37–46.

Stocker, M. and Hegeman, E. (1996) *Valuing Emotions*. Melbourne: Cambridge University Press.

Summers-Effler, E. (2002) The Micro Potential for Social Change: Emotion, Consciousness, and Social Movement Formation. *Sociological Theory* 20: 41–60.

Surbone, A. (2006) Cultural Aspects of Communication in Cancer Care. In: Stiefel, F. (ed.). *Communication in Cancer Care*. Berlin: Springer.

Sweeting, H.N. and Gilhooly, M.L. (1990) Anticipatory Grief: A Review. *Social Science & Medicine* 30: 1,073–80.

Szollos, A. (2009) Toward a Psychology of Chronic Time Pressure: Conceptual and Methodological Review. *Time and Society* 18: 332–50.

Szreter, S. (2002) Rethinking McKeown: the Relationship Between Public Health and Social Change. *American Journal of Public Health* 92: 722–5.

Taylor, S., Foster, M. and Flemming, J. (2008) *Health Care Practice in Australia: Policy, Context and Innovations*. South Melbourne: Oxford University Press.

Taylor, S.E. and Dakof, G.A. (1988) Social Support and the Cancer Patient. In: Spacapan, S. and Oskamp, S. (eds). *The Social Psychology of Health*. London: Sage Publications, 95–116.

The World Bank. (2014) *Life Expectancy at Birth, Total (years)*. Washington, DC: The World Bank.

Thomas, C. and Morris, S.M. (2002) Informal Carers in Cancer Contexts. *European Journal of Cancer Care* 11: 178–82.

Thomas, C., Morris, S.M. and Harman, J.C. (2002) Companions Through Cancer: the Care Given by Informal Carers in Cancer Contexts. *Social Science & Medicine* 54: 529–44.

Thomas, C., Morris, S.M, Soothill, K., et al. (2001) *What are the psychosocial needs of cancer patients and their main carers? A study of user experiences of cancer services with particular reference to psychosocial need*. Lancaster: The Institute for Health Research, Lancaster University.

Thompson, E.H. (2005) What's Unique About Men's Caregiving? In: Kramer, B.J. and Thompson, E.H.J. (eds). *Men as Caregivers*. Amherst, NY: Prometheus Books, 20–47.

Tomarken, A., Holland, J., Schachter, S., et al. (2008) Factors of Complicated Grief Pre-Death in Caregivers of Cancer Patients. *Psycho-oncology* 17: 105–11.

Toscano, N. (2014) Minimum Wage Up 3 Per Cent, Rise of $18.70 a Week. *The Sydney Morning Herald*. Sydney: Fairfax Media.

Toseland, R., Blanchard, C. and McCallion, P. (1995) A Problem Solving Intervention for Caregivers of Cancer Patients. *Social Science & Medicine* 40: 517–28.

Tovey, P., Chatwin, J. and Broom, A. (2007) *Traditional, Complementary and Alternative Medicine and Cancer Care*. London: Routledge.

Tsilika, E., Mystakidou, K., Parpa, E., et al. (2009) The Influence of Cancer Impact On Patients' Preparatory Grief. *Psychology and Health* 24: 135–48.

Turner, B.S. (2006) Hospital. *Theory, Culture & Society* 23: 573–9.

Turner, J.H. and Stets, J.E. (2005) *The Sociology of Emotions*. New York: Cambridge University Press.

Twigg, J. and Atkin, K. (1994) *Carers Perceived: Policy and Practice in Informal Care*. Buckingham: Open University Press.

Ugalde, A., Krishnasamy, M. and Schofield, P. (2012) Role Recognition and Changes to Self-Identity in Family Caregivers of People with Advanced Cancer: A Qualitative Study. *Support Care Cancer* 20: 1,175–81.

Ussher, J. and Sandoval, M. (2008) Gender Differences in the Construction and Experience of Cancer Care: The Consequences of the Gendered Positioning of Carers. *Psychology and Health* 23: 945–63.

Waldrop, D.P. (2007) Caregiver Grief in Terminal Illness and Bereavement: A Mixed-Methods Study. *Health & Social Work* 32: 197–206.

Weicht, B. (2011) Embracing Dependency: Rethinking (in)Dependence in the Discourse of Care. *The Sociological Review* 58: 205–24.

Weitzner, M.A., Haley, W.E. and Chen, H. (2000) The Family Caregiver of the Older Cancer Patient. *Hematology/oncology Clinics of North America* 14: 269–81.

Wharton, A.S. (2009) The Sociology of Emotional Labor. *Annual Review of Sociology* 35: 147–65.

Wharton, A.S. and Erickson, R.J. (1995) The Consequences of Caring: Exploring the Links Between Women's Job and Family Emotion Work. *Sociological Quarterly* 36: 273–96.

White, K. (2006) *Sage Dictionary of Health and Society*. London: Sage Publications.

Whiting, P. and James, E. (2006) *Bearing witness to the story: Narrative reconstruction in grief counseling*. Alexandria, VA: American Counseling Association.

Wilkinson, A. (2006) Caregiving. *Women's Health Seminar Series*. Bethesda, MD.

Wilkinson, S. and Kitzinger, C. (2000) Thinking Differently About Thinking Positive: A Discursive Approach to Cancer Patients' Talk. *Social Science & Medicine* 50: 797–811.

Williams, J.K., Skirton, H., Paulsen, J.S., et al. (2009) The Emotional Experiences of Family Carers in Huntington Disease. *Journal of Advanced Nursing* 65: 789–98.

Wolkomir, M. (2001) Emotion Work, Commitment, and the Authentication of the Self. *Journal of Contemporary Ethnography* 30: 305–34.

Woof, R. and Nyatanga, B. (1998) Adapting to Death, Dying, and Bereavement. In: Faull, C., Carter, Y. and Woof, R. (eds). *Handbook of Palliative Care*. Carlton, VIC: Blackwell Science, Ltd, 74–87.

Wright, A.A., Zhang, B., Ray, A., et al. (2008) Associations Between End-of-Life Discussions, Patient Mental Health, Medical Care Near Death, and Caregiver Bereavement Adjustment. *Journal of the American Medical Association* 300: 1,665–73.

Wyatt, S., Harris, R. and Wathen, N. (2010) Health(y) Citizenship: Technology, Work and Narratives of Responsibility. In: Harris, R., Wathen, N. and Wyatt, S. (eds). *Configuring Health Consumers: Health Work and the Imperative of Personal Responsibility*. New York: Palgrave Macmillan, 1–10.

Zapf, D. (2002) Emotion Work and Psychological Well-Being: A Review of the Literature and Some Conceptual Considerations. *Human Resource Management Review* 12: 237–68.

Zarit, S., Todd, P. and Zarit, J. (1986) Subjective Burden of Husbands and Wives as Caregivers: A Longitudinal Study. *The Gerontologist* 26: 260–66.

Zimmerman, C. (2007) Death Denial: Obstacle or Instrument for Palliative Care? An Analysis of Clinical Literature. *Sociology of Health & Illness* 29: 297–314.

Appendix A
Interview Guide for Initial Interviews[1]

What type of cancer does your partner have?

How long have you been providing support for him/her?

What role do you see yourself playing in his/her care?

Starting from the beginning and in as much detail as possible, tell me about your experiences or overall story of being a carer.

What would ideal support be? What would the ideal service provider do?

What kind of care/support would you have liked?

What do you think and feel about your experiences as a carer?

Who supports you and how?

What do you think about support groups?

How do you deal with the emotional side of being a carer?

What role did medical and support service personnel play in how you dealt with the emotional side of being a carer?

What would you say your biggest needs are?

1 These interview guides were originally published by John Wiley & Sons Ltd: Olson, R.E. (2014c). Indefinite Loss: The Experiences of Carers of a Spouse with Carer. *European Journal of Cancer Care* 23(4): 553–61. http://onlinelibrary.wiley.com/enhanced/doi/10.1111/ecc.12175/.

Appendix B
Interview Guide for Follow-up Interviews

Last time we talked you told me … [summarise main points of their story].

How are you feeling about this now?

Who supports you and how?

What do you think about support groups?

What would you say your biggest needs are?

How do you deal with the emotional side of being a carer?

Do you feel uncertain about what emotions you should be feeling as a carer and spouse?

Do you ever self-censor?

Do you feel appreciated/valued as a husband/wife carer?

What role does time play in your experience as a carer?

Did you feel our discussion last time had an impact on how you think or feel about being a carer/spouse for someone with cancer?

What has changed over the past six months?

Index

Printed and bound by CPI Group (UK) Ltd, Croydon, CR0 4YY

24/10/2024

01778283-0019